THE CROWNING TOUCH

Preparing for Beauty Pageant Competition

by Anna Stanley

BOX OF IDEAS PUBLISHING, SAN DIEGO

This book is dedicated to every girl who has ever entered a pageant of mine. It has been wonderful working with so many real winners.

Published by Box of Ideas Publishing
P.O. Box 1648
San Diego, Ca 92118

Library of Congress Cataloging-in-Publication Data

Stanley, Anna.
  The Crowining Touch.

  1. Beauty pageants — United States — Handbooks, manuals, etc. I. Stanley, Anna. II. Title.
                                                            89-60857
ISBN 0-9621972-1-1

Manufactured in the United States of America

10 9 8 7 6 5 4 3 2 1

First Edition

Acknowledgements

This book would not have been possible without the research assistance of Karen Kemple and the polishing editiorial and organizational skills of Nitalu Sroka. To them I owe my heartfelt gratitude for seeing this project through.

Acknowledgements

Table of Contents

3 - APPEARANCE: GROOMING TECHNIQUES

4 - POLISHING YOUR COMPETITIVE PERSONA

5 - The Pageant and Beyond   93

- Appendix A   113

- Appendix B   114

- Appendix C   121

*To be born woman is to know — although they
do not talk of it at school — that we must
labour to be beautiful.*

—*William Butler Yeats*

Chapter 1

SO YOU WANT TO BECOME A BEAUTY QUEEN

Like many girls, you have dreamed of winning a pageant. Walking down a runway with a crown on your head is a dream that can become reality if you really want it and apply yourself. Just remember that most pageants are not really "beauty" pageants. They are contests for girls with poise and personality. With this in mind and a winning attitude, you are sure to be a winner.

There are many reasons why girls enter pageants. For most girls, their aspirations are to become a high-paid model and actress. Entering a pageant allows a girl to gain visibility. For Courtney Gibbs, *Miss USA* 1988, her hopes were that pageants would lead her to a career in broadcasting. (She was already a professional model when she entered the *Miss USA* system.)

Annually, millions of girls enter pageants to derive the benefits of competing. For many, participating in pageants gives them self-confidence and teaches them poise. It forces them to prove they are "genuine" — not the stereotyped image of a pretty-but-phony beauty queen. Pageants offer them insight into how well-prepared they are to face life, with or without that ultimate crown. Very few girls become *Miss America*, but what's wrong with success on a local or regional scale. Success, after all, is being happy with where you are and what you are doing.

Pageants are good for helping girls to overcome shyness.

Everyone realizes it takes willpower to fight shyness, so those of you who are shy are to be commended for entering your first pageant. Kelli Lee, *Miss South Texas Teen* 1985, did not overcome shyness for her first pageant, but used her first pageant to determine whether or not she wished to continue competing. "The fact that I was shy was the reason for entering the pageant and from there I had to decide whether or not i wanted to be less shy and meet other people. Overcoming shyness comes with continued exposure."

Another benefit of being a part of pageant competition is the opportunities it offers you. Kathi Eidsmoe, a San Diego pageant contestant, feels that competition forces her to evaluate herself. Kelli Lee feels " ... every competition is a learning experience and I feel growth from each pageant. Each competition leaves me feeling more 'in tune' to myself. Whether it comes during the training time, during the pageant itself or afterward during an evaluation of my performance, more knowledge about myself is gained." *Pageant Review* suggests other potential benefits of pageant competition:

- Career opportunities
- Gaining confidence and determination
- Learning to set goals and achieve them
- Learning positive ways to react under stress
- Learning to speak in public
- Learning to find and develop your best assets
- Learning poise and testing it under stress
- Learning how to receive constructive criticism
- Developing a sense of competition for future life situations
- Learning how to present yourself onstage
- Learning to win and lose gracefully

Pageants encourage women to "reach their full potential and be all that they can be," says *Miss California* 1988, Marlise Sharleen Ricardo. Pageants teach women to project a professional image that allows them to get ahead while at the same time learning to be physically attractive.

Meeting people who share your interest is another benefit of entering pageants. You love entering pageants, chances are so do they. You'll have a lot in common. Other benefits include exposure to new things and the opportunity to travel to new places. According to Kelli Lee, the nice thing about entering pageants is "definitely the people that you meet. I have friends all over the U.S. that I have made through pageants. However, I do not only consider the contestants as friends, I look forward to meeting the directors and the professional people connected with the pageants. I have had the privilege of working with top Hollywood directors and stars as a result of pageants."

Girls enter pageants so they can learn to market their future businesses. Mary Elizabeth Haroth, *Miss Maryland* 1984, a 25-year-old dental student, entered pageants to learn how to market her future practice through positive public relations.

For Kelli Lee, pageants have strengthened her and taught her how to handle rejection as well as success, thereby allowing her to handle that aspect of the entertainment business. "Even if a girl is not inclined toward the 'business,' I feel that the interview portion of pageant competition prepares a girl for job interviews, scholarship interviews and meeting people in general."

Psychological, Social, and Emotional Benefits of Looking Beautiful

Looking beautiful has psychological, social, and emotional benefits. Self-enhancement improves the way others see you and respond to you, improving your relationships with them. More importantly, looking good improves your self-image and self-esteem. If you know you look good, you begin to feel better about yourself. With a little outward confidence in your appearance comes a whole new inner confidence in your intelligence.

Pageants are good for girls because they usually motivate them to improve themselves. Pageants give girls confidence and teach them determination and responsibility, allowing them to develop their personality. Pageant coach Mary Francis Flood advises, "Participation in a pageant definitely teaches a girl determination and responsibility. You do not necessarily need that prior to entering a pageant. It can be developed." Contestants learn to present one look — their most beautiful one.

Pageantry as a Vehicle for Building Confidence

Many pageants attract contestant by presenting pageantry as a vehicle for building confidence. In this context, prizes are viewed as the "icing on the cake." This rewarding experience is cited by pageant winners and is the result of a new respectability in pageants. Contestants soon learn that pageants are not simply beauty contests. The prettiest girl does not always win. They soon find that judges and pageant officials stress poise, speaking ability, goals, and an amiable personality as essential ingredients for a winner. Actually, it is the survival of the fittest mentally. It is the most humbling experience contestants go through. They learn what they're made of. They learn to reach down and really pull from inside. "To have true beauty, a girl needs to possess many qualities: belief in herself, a commitment to herself, humility and the ability to accept defeat as a challenge," advises Mary Francis Flood. While judges put great emphasis on the whole girl, at the same time, they want every detail about her to be perfect.

Life is a continuous competition in various degrees. Be good sports and accept defeat as a challenge and success with humility. Realize that you are your greatest competitor and do not be intimidated by others. Only compete with yourself, pushing yourself to your own limits. Then be happy with that. If you waste time sizing up your competition, then you take away from your own energy, possibly cheating yourself of having been the very best you could have been. Preparation is the best intimidation. Laura Martinez Herring, *Miss USA* 1985, says, "If you spend too much time worrying about the contestant next to you having longer legs, prettier teeth, or a better figure, you will detract from your own self." The moment you start worrying about how good or bad you are compared to another, jealousy or pride are sure to creep in to distract you. Wearing a crown is not nearly as important as how you make it shine.

Scholarship Pageants

According to an article in *The San Diego Union*, pageant officials at the *Miss California* pageant say that, through scholarships, the pageant offers participants the opportunity to further their education. Officials note that judging is based on talent, poise and the ability to communicate — in addition, to beauty. Robert Arnhm, president of the *Miss California* pageant, notes, "We have some very bright women involved here." The *Miss California* pageant began in 1921, but along the way, times have changed. The *Miss America* pageant is no longer seeking a bathing beauty. *Miss California* 1988, Marlise Sharleen Ricardos, notes about her experience, "It is not a beauty contest. It is a scholarship pageant. This will help me attain studies that I would otherwise not be able to afford." She added that it was the scholarship money that had motivated her to become involved in beauty pageants. "Every time you enter a program, each contestant receives a scholarship, so no one walks away a loser."

Miss America and other national pageant systems have certainly helped lots of women further their education and develop opportunities that would have been unavailable otherwise.

It Takes More Than Lady Luck to Win a Beauty Pageant

Many girls, especially first time contenders, don't take pageants seriously because they don't know what to expect. To most, appearance and luck seem to be the important aspects. Little do they know that there are so many more qualities that go along with being a winner. It takes more than Lady Luck to win a beauty pageant.

Saying "Beauty and Brains Don't Mix" is Out of Date

The old saying "beauty and brains don't mix" is simply out of date. The fact is, girls who feel smart usually enjoy looking smart. According to an article in the *Los Angeles Time*, you rarely see the prom queen interested in science, because "it's not considered feminine." What is unfeminine about being smart? Many contestants excel in academics, including science. Christy Cole, a former titleholder and a Texas pageant coach, received her master's degree in science. America will accept a smart beauty queen, so don't settle for being less than you can be. Women have more to offer than skin-deep beauty. A pageant can be a magical time for most contestants, putting them into "the pageantry trance." During this "magical" time, do not forget about the significance of good grades and a good education. Keep your grades up.

What Type of Girl Wins Beauty Pageants

Girls often ask what type of girl is most likely to win a beauty pageant. It is not the girl who has the most expensive wardrobe or sophisticated appearance that can win over the judges. Many judges see these girls as fake and are not impressed. It's not always the prettiest girl. A contestant who is blessed with good looks and talent may not have the temperament to be a beauty queen. The girls who best typify the American ideal of charm, personality, perfect grooming, and fresh good looks, as well as show their intellect *are* the natural and sincere ones. Beauty depends a great deal on good judgment. A winner has to have B.B.'s (beauty and brains). A girl cannot possess one without the other and be a winner. She must also be tireless and capable of making endless personal appearances. The girl who wins a pageant is the girl who is competing because she wants to, not because someone else wants it for her. According to Ieda Maria Vargas, *Miss Universe* 1963, the recipe for a winner is simple: "The most important thing is a cup full of good attitude, then add yourself, do not fake your personality or your appearance, nor be cynical about life. Add another cup of virtue and intellect. Mix them up in a large international bowl and let the judges make the decision of what the mold should be."[1]

"Probably the most important quality a contestant must possess in order to be a winner is that of self-confidence," advises Kelli Lee. "Believe in yourself, and other will believe in you." Self-confident people radiate power, success and health. Others want to be just like them. For those who lack self-confidence, it is a skill that can be practiced. people tend to confuse self-confidence with egotism. The key is being confident without being conceited. A contestant who is self-confident in a interview will make the judges feel confident. Be confident in yourself, otherwise no one will be confident in you.

Persistence Pays

Persistence pays. If a contestant keeps learning from her experience and doesn't give up — even competing in a different preliminary, she may prevail. The proof stands in the story of

---

1   Ana Maria Cumba, *The World of Miss Universe*, Manyland Books, Inc.

Debra Sue Maffett, *Miss America* 1983. Debra competed in the *Miss Texas* pageant on three occasions, making the top 10 on her first attempt, 2nd runner-up on her second and 4th runner-up on her third try. She then entered the *Miss Texas USA* pageant, finishing as 2nd runner-up on her first attempt and 3rd runner-up her next. She then moved to California and won the *Miss Anaheim* pageant, the *Miss California* pageant, and the *Miss America* pageant.

Phyllis George and Shirley Cothran are symbols of tenacity and grace under pressure. Both women lost their first pageants — Phyllis to a drummer, Shirley to a roller skater — before winning the *Miss America* title.

One advantage of recompeting in a pageant is that you know the ropes. After one unsuccessful pageant attempt, you'll know more about yourself and have a better idea of how to impress the judges. "Every time you compete you learn more about yourself, become more poised, polished and self-confident," notes Texas pageant director Karen Kemple. Phyllis George, *Miss America* 1971, was first runner-up in the *Miss Texas* pageant the year before she won it, eventually winning the national crown. Contestants are more at ease the second time around. The only drawback to this is they also risk becoming plastic. Some contestants may forget how to come across as sincere. Judges find it obvious that they're hearing something the contestant thinks they want to hear.

Success Stories

Mary Johanna Harum, now better known as Mary Hart, co-host of "Entertainment Tonight," says pageants were a part of her childhood dreams that became a reality. She represented South Dakota in the *Miss America* pageant. Though she had lots of fun, she admitted it was a lot of pressure. She learned to be competitive and has always been glad to have competed. For Mary Hart, pageants provided a way to develop her skills. The interview taught her to express herself verbally, learning that *how* you say something is as important as *what* you say. Realizing the importance of poise and carriage allowed her to become aware of her inner self and self-confident in front of an audience. Most importantly, it spurred her on to become a TV talk host.

Phyllis George was able to fulfill her ambition of being a

television broadcaster when she was hired by CBS for their NFL sports program. Phyllis credits her beauty pageant title with being very helpful to her career. "I made a lot of money during my year's reign with promotions and appearances (about $150,000). It just opened up all kinds of doors for me, especially through the traveling I did during the year, meeting so many interesting and important people. I had led a very quiet life until that year, and it just opened up a whole new world for me at the age of twenty-one. I would say it's a type of show-biz — it gave me confidence and the title was influential in my career."[2]

Kathryn Crosby, who started as *Splash Day Princess* at age three, went on to become *Rodeo Queen of the Fatstock Show,* as well as first runner-up for *Miss Texas.* "Women's Lib hasn't changed my feelings about beauty contests at all. In fact, it was a form of liberation for me. I learned to make speeches, to compete, and to meet all types of people."[3]

Lindsay Diane Bloom, who plays opposite Stacy Keach as Mike Hammer's witty secretary, has said her pageant experience gave her a wonderful opportunity to show her talents. They taught her how to get along with people and how to accept and handle competition. She also learned how to handle interviews with the judges and the press. She had such a desire for a career and felt that pageants were the only way anyone was going to see her talent. Her four years of pageant experience taught her poise, how to speak in public, how to interview, self-confidence and how to handle pressure.

Kim Bassinger credits pageants with helping her overcome her insecurities. She had agoraphobia and was home-bound for months. One day she forced herself into the spotlight and into the *Junior Miss* pageant. For the talent competition, she sang "Wouldn't It Be Loverly" from *My Fair Lady.* She had worked on it for weeks, but was terrified. She didn't care about winning; she just wanted to get through the performance without passing out. That night, she did it flawlessly, brilliantly! To her, that was the best performance she had ever given. "You could've heard a pin

2   Marie Fenton Griffing, *How to Be a Beauty Pageant Winner,* Fireside books.
3   *San Francisco Chronicle,* May 10, 1976.

drop. Everybody in high school who ever thought I never said three words couldn't believe it. I won."[4]

Areas of Competition

In pageants, the areas of competition are as varied as the pageants themselves. The *National College Queen* pageant includes skills such as cake decorating, highway and safety practices, and color coordination in their eleven judging criteria. The *Maid of Cotton* pageant requires finalists to make a two minute speech about why they would like to be the *Maid*. San Francisco's *Miss Chinatown USA* contestants were once required to answer on-stage questions in Chinese. Audiences did not hesitate to laugh if a contestant's Chinese was not up to par. Some pageants single out particular features or characteristics in their criteria. Some single out the most beautiful hands, feet, legs, hair, figure and face; others require contestants to demonstrate their personality, manners and graciousness while dining with the judges. Because of its special cultural heritage, Jamaica decided to select ten queens in celebration of its 300th year under British rule. To recognize the racial diversity of the island, categories were set up by the racial ancestry and/or skin coloring of the contestants.

Chapter 2

MAJOR AREAS OF COMPETITION

The Interview

The most important category in any pageant is the interview. It is the opportunity for the judges to evaluate personality and general awareness. Pageants are won and lost in the interview. A girl can be an idiot and photogenic, but a beauty queen must be intelligent. Karen Kemple notes, "If you are in a close race with another, the girl who has the better interview will probably win."

At the same time, Karen remarks, "The judges are there because they want to meet you, not to try to scare you or trick you with questions." You should not be afraid of them. If anything, the interview should be a fun experience. It is a chance to sit down and talk with community leaders, successful business people and celebrities. If you can overcome your initial fright before you step into the interview room, you will have won half of the battle. If you impress the judges in the interview, they will *want* to like you in other areas of competition. On the other hand, pageant coach Mary Francis Flood warns, "If you come across as an inexperienced or poor interviewer, you might as well hang it up. You really have to have a good interview. You need to have your own opinion on things, not another's. You need to learn to think on your feet."

The judges' interview is really a forum. It offers the judges an opportunity to observe how a girl expresses herself and how she carries off a difficult moment. The trick is to have stamina and presence, to look confident and be comfortable. To master this, you must learn to really listen. Don't be flustered and anticipate what you THINK will be asked. This is your opportunity to demonstrate your stamina, grace and ability to field the unexpected — the very traits the titleholder will have to demonstrate during the hectic year of her reign.

The Proper Way to Enter the Interview Room

Enter the interview room with good posture, with excitement and enthusiasm, controlled energy, and a friendly smile. Go into your interview confident that you are going to like your interview and the judges. "You should be excited that the judges are going to have a chance to meet you and see you and hear from you. The look forward to that," notes Jane Jaffe, instructor at John Robert Powers. Barbara Kelley, former *Miss Virginia* and director of "The Winning Look" seminars, advises, "just like the Boy Scouts, you must be prepared." Greet the judges when you enter the interview room. You may greet them in many ways, using this as an ice breaker. If you are meeting the judges one-on-one, a handshake is ideal, but if you are being judged by a panel, it can become awkward. A poised, simple "Hello" is also fine. In either case, wait to be offered a seat.

Pageant interviews are like job interviews. "I looked at the whole thing as a job interview. You think about the company and what its needs are. You try to put yourself in their shoes. If you don't understand their needs, then you're not going to do a good job for them," says *Miss American Petite* 1988 Stephanie Raye. When a contestant enters a pageant, she is applying for a job. She should not go into a job interview unprepared, and the same applies to pageant competition. Approach the pageant interview on a professional level. When preparing for interview questions, consider a variety of questions that may be asked and think about how you would respond to them. Although you should be natural and relaxed in the interview, it is difficult to feel this way if you are not prepared. Mock interviews or practicing with friends will help you prepare for the real thing.

Creating the First Impression

Self-confidence radiates from the girl who walks into the interview knowing that she has the skills and knowledge to handle the pageant title and its responsibilities. Make your sparkling eyes speak to the judges. Do not stare at the floor or the wall behind the judges. On the other hand, don't constantly move your eyes up and down the line of judges. Instead, gracefully move from one judge to another in no particular order like you would when speaking to a group of people at a social gathering. Relaxed eye contact shows your confidence and command of the situation. Due to time limitations, some judges may not have the opportunity to ask you a question. Having made relaxed, confident eye contact with these judges may be your only opportunity to establish a bond.

Debra Sue Maffett, *Miss America* 1983, remembers, "A contestant's first interview with the judges is very intense. It's the first time a judge sees you, and they form an impression that lasts through the contest. Maybe it's not supposed to, but that's human nature."[1] You only get one chance to make a first impression! At the same time, judges have no one with whom to compare their first contestant. Therefore, "it is most important that you make a lasting impression so that your interview does not fade in their memories during the remainder of the interviews," advises Karen Kemple. Judges tend to remember those they have interviewed most recently unless they have been strongly impressed. In both the *Miss California* and *Miss America* pageants, Debra Sue Maffett won the title after having been one of the first contestants interviewed — it can be done.

During the Interview

During the interview, you should speak confidently and emphasize your strengths. Cheryl Prewitt-Salem, *Miss America* 1980, advises, "Always 'sell' yourself. No one else is going to do that for you. No one else cares as much about you — your plans, goals and dreams — as you do. Always build yourself up."

Christy Cole has many good suggestions for the interview. "I know it may seem virtually impossible to not be nervous, but you should do your best to hide it if possible." Take your time before answering a question. "This doesn't mean waiting ten minutes to

1   *San Francisco Chronicle*, July 4, 1982

answer! When asked a question, pause for a moment and select your thoughts and words carefully. Learn to organize your thoughts before starting to speak. Then take a breath before answering. This gives your brain a few more seconds to think about what it will say before it comes out of your mouth. Do not feel this will make you look indecisive; it only lets them know you are seriously considering the question. This also helps to eliminate saying words like: well-a, aaa, and 'That's a hard/good question.' Never admit out loud to the judges that the question is hard — that's why they asked it! Do not try to change the subject in the middle of your answer. Nine times out of ten this ends up in disaster. I might add that if a contestant is asked a question about something she has never heard of, she should not quit smiling." On the other hand, "If the line of questioning is leading nowhere, try to regain control of the conversation and lead into a positive area. Do not, nevertheless, try to take over the entire interview!"

When it comes to demeanor in the interview, Christy has still other suggestions to offer. "Never should you rest both arms on an interview chair. One arm is acceptable, lightly resting, not clutching, but never both." Similarly avoid speaking with your hands. "If you gesture with your hands, then you are not answering the question properly. Besides, hands that flit constantly are distracting. Clasp both hands together in your lap. This allows you to squeeze your fingers together and prevent that ever-present handshaking that goes along with nervousness! This will also remove the urge to talk with your hands." Ideally, your hands will rest together in your lap, palms upward, in a controlled manner that suggests openness. Do not play with your fingernails, rings, or anything else that can reveal your nervousness.

Judges Have Reasons for Asking Specific Questions

Remember, judges have reasons for asking specific questions. The manner in which you answer can be more important than the content of your answer. What matters in the interview is not what you know, it's the impression you make on the judges. Some questions will be designed to see if you have depth or if you just have sawdust; others will be silly to see if you will give an interesting, intelligent answer. Still other questions will be thought provoking or even unanswerable. Whatever questions you field, Barbara Kelley advises, "remember the KISS method:

Keep it short and sweet." At the same time, avoid making your answer so brief that the judges feel they haven't learned anything about you.

"... if you do not know the answer [to a question], do not try to fake it and answer incorrectly. You may accidentally get the right answer, but the odds are much greater that you won't," says Christy Cole. "I might also add, the judges will go a lot easier on a girl who admits her limitations, rather than a girl who makes her ignorance 'hard to ignore.' If a judge asks you a question you cannot answer, simply say 'I'm sorry, I don't know.' There is nothing wrong with you admitting you don't know everything." As a matter of fact, *Miss America* judge Nanci Wudel admits, "I often ask a question that I know they can't answer just to get their reaction."

If you encounter a question that you can't answer, count on your personality to save the day. When Deborah Mosley, *Miss Georgia* 1978, was asked her opinion of then U.S. Representative Barbara Jordan, she didn't know who she way. She responded, I don't know who she is, but just as soon as this interview is over, I'm going to find out."

Be Prepared for Possible Questions

Be prepared for many possible interview questions. If it is an election year, be well informed on local and national candidates and issues. Having an educated awareness of your region makes it easier to be an effective representative — after all, that is part of the job of a titleholder. By all means, know the names of the President, the Vice-President, and the Secretary of State, as well as those of the Governor or your state, the Mayor of your city, and any important personages associated with your pageant. In the 1982 *Miss America* pageant, *Miss Texas* thought she had done well in the interview. She had known the answer to all but one of her questions. "What was the question?" asked B. Don Magness, director of the *Miss Texas* pageant. "The question was 'Who is Albert Marks?'" came the reply. At that time, Mr. Marks was the chairman of the board of the *Miss America* pageant[2].

2   *San Francisco Chronicle*, September 16, 1982

Showing Your Sense of Humor

Humor is a good indication of the confidence level among people. Showing your sense of humor when appropriate, therefore, can make a good impression on the judges. For example, to avoid appearing too opinionated, you might field a question about the U.S. economy by quipping, "I would give anything if our dollar would go a little farther." At the same time, the caveat when appropriate is important. If the question is of a serious nature, Texas pageant director and coach Donna Lee comments, "I do not feel that the contestant should keep a plastic smile glued on her face — that makes her appear 'stupid.' If the situation warrants a smile, then it should be there."

Never Repeat the Question

Never repeat the question before answering it. Repeating the question does not give you more time to think; it indicates that you are nervous. Similarly, "I'm glad you asked that question" is trite and creates the wrong impression. When you are asked a question, pause and silently compose your answer. Do not give cliche answers or respond with the first thought that comes to mind. For example, if you are asked why you entered this pageant, there are both trivial and thoughtful responses. Citing personal development, gaining poise, self-pride and career opportunities creates a much better impression than saying "to have fun and make friends."

Toward the end of your interview, a judge may ask you if there is anything you would like to ask the panel. Be prepared for this by having several potential questions in mind. You will appear confident, comfortable and in control. Possible questions to demonstrate your sincere interest in them might include "What are you seeking in a winner?", "Do you enjoy being a judge?", "What is the most difficult part of judging?", "Have you judged this pageant before?" If the timer bell rings in the middle of your answer, finish responding, unless you are told to do otherwise, but make your response brief.

Concluding the Interview

To conclude the interview, stand up, smile at each judge, thank them and leave. Barbara Kelley warns, "Don't be 'adorable' by saying 'Oh, it's over? It went so fast!'" Once out of the interview room do not discuss your interview with other contestants. This is a contest, however friendly, and you do not want them to have the unfair advantage of extra time to prepare their answers.

Preparing for the Interview Competition

The best way to prepare for your interview is to study and practice. This will not only allow you to be prepared for a larger variety of questions, it will also help you conquer nervousness. Many times the judges' interview questions come from the entry application. Therefore, an ideal way to prepare for this area of competition is to turn every item on your application into a question and practice composing answers.

Deborah Mosley, *Miss Georgia* 1978, videotaped mock interviews with the news staff of WRBL-TV. She then played the tape to see what flaws needed correcting. This technique is useful to catch such fatal flaws as nervous laughter. If the giggles start to intrude, take a deep breath, slowly exhale, and proceed to your thought-provoking answer. You, too, can approach your favorite news station and ask that they judge you in a taped mock interview. Most will be happy to assist you in achieving your goal. They may also use their video recorder to tape the interview, as well as take the time to go over your tape, helping you correct flaws.

Debra Sue Maffett, *Miss America* 1983, felt that reading helped her capture her crown. She studied sociology, psychology and current events. She says she learned a lot and was ready for any question the judges asked.

Frequently Asked Questions

Another way to build confidence and conquer nerves is to practice interview techniques with family and friends. Repeatedly answering spontaneous questions will help you overcome shyness. Practice interviews can make you more comfortable with any question a journalist or pageant judge might ask. (A list of typical pageant interview questions is in Appendix B.) Barbara Kelley has written a two volume book of pageant questions. Volume I has 286 of the most frequently asked interview questions. Volume II has 206 completely different questions. These questions are sorted by categories, such as Psychological, Opinion, Social, Moral, Political, Religious, Self-evaluation, Analytical, Current Events Questions, and Questions arising from contestant questionnaires.

When asked a question such as "What makes you feel important," Barbara comments under self-evaluation questions, "Is it the clubs or organizations you belong to, your hobbies, the number of dates you have each weekend, the number of invitations you get to parties, compliments about your clothes, or even a physical feature? Perhaps it's a major weight loss, your G.P.A., your pageant accomplishments, or the car you drive. When you determine the origin of your self-esteem, you'll know a lot more about your priorities and values. You might discover that you're materialistic — and that's not all bad, as long as you're willing to work hard (school or job) to put yourself in the financial position to afford the things you like. If it's clubs, organizations, or hobbies, you may discover they're leading to a career path. Whatever the case, the things that make you feel important are where you direct your energies. Accomplishment in the areas reinforces your self-esteem. When you give an answer to this question, back it up with why it makes you feel important and how it fits into your life-goals — if it does. Maybe it just makes you feel good! If that's the case, tell why."

A typical question under the category religion would be "What do you want most from a religious organization?" Barbara analyzes possible answers to this by commenting, "A standard answer would be salvation, spiritual growth or an extended family. You could give more depth to your response by considering some of the following: encouragement and uplifting, self-improvement, ceremonial support for weddings/funerals, and singing of hymns or Christian music that's vibrant and uplifting. At one pageant, a contestant said, 'A lot of people act as if the Ten Commandments were the 10 Suggestions, so I want sermons with a stronger emphasis put on the scriptures. So many sermons today are more like motivational talks.'" See Appendix C for information about ordering Barbara Kelley's books.

Since many pageant judges ask the same basic questions, scripting well thought-out replies ahead of time will raise your comfort and confidence level, thereby increasing your chances of winning the title. Below are some frequently asked questions — with possible answers — to help you prepare.

1. *Tell me about yourself.* What you say about yourself is the single most important factor in any interview. You can literally talk yourself into — or out of — a title. What the judges really want to know is what you can do for the pageant and why you should be selected the Queen over the other contestants. Simply outline several of your strong points and accomplishments. When you've listed these, make a summary statement and then stop talking.

Interviewers generally will ask you questions about yourself. Relax and enjoy the subject; no one knows you better than you do. Practice answering questions about your hobbies, ambitions, why you entered the pageant, why you want to be the winner, etc. Rehearsing answers beforehand allows you to field these questions confidently when the time comes. Always answer enthusiastically, and never put yourself down. Jane Jaffe says, "Most girls don't know themselves because they haven't prepared by asking themselves, 'Who am I?'" When Jane serves on a judging panel, the first question she asks is "Tell me about yourself." If you are asked this question, do not respond with the items that are on your application. The judges probably have that in front of them. Tell them something they do not know. Jane warns, "If you give information to judges that is already in front of them, you're wasting your precious time. You only have a few minutes to impress the judges. If you're not telling them anything new, you're not impressing them."

2. *What qualifies you for the title?* Always mention your most impressive qualifications first. Your opening line is frequently what really registers with an interviewer. In addition, prepare some success stories ahead of time, then drop them casually into your answer as if they were spontaneous thought. For example, "Dedicating an entire year in preparing for this pageant qualifies me for the title." Giving an answer such as this one shows your interviewer that you've worked hard in a positive direction to be

where you are and that you don't plan on stopping. He or she will think that you're the right girl for the title, after all.

3. *Why did you enter this pageant?* Avoid answers like "for the prize package offered" or "to travel." These sound frivolous. Instead, show that you've done some homework on the pageant and what it represents by giving an answer that reflects the goal of the pageant. For example, if you know the pageant is involved with the "Just Say No" program, your answer could be "To support the 'Just Say No' program in any way I can. I am glad this pageant is offering me the opportunity to do just that."

4. *What are your weaknesses?* This sounds like a trick question, but it is actually quite easy to answer. The "best" weaknesses are disguised strengths, such as "I dislike it when I'm unchallenged by my work" or "Sometimes I get too involved with a project and don't have time to visit with my friends." With this latter answer, they'll see that you're the type of person they are seeking to represent the title precisely because your friends *won't* distract you from your responsibilities.

5. *What are your strengths?* Your recital should highlight the qualities that will help you succeed as the titleholder. For example, determination, a persuasive personality, friendliness, and the ability to analyze people quickly are all traits that would be positive for a titleholder to possess.

6. *What is unique about you?* Many young girls have not lived long enough to have really figured out who they are, what they are or what they're about. When Jane Jaffe asks a contestant "What is unique about you?", contestants often respond "Well, nothing." That's not true. Every one of us is unique and special. Find out what's unique about yourself by taking a survey. "Maybe it's not your eyes, your hair and you skin. Maybe it's the difference in the genuineness of your soul. Maybe you really are a friendly person. Maybe you are that caring and compassionate girl who cares about other people. That's what you have to find out," says Jane Jaffe. "That's where your confidence will come from when you realize you have something special to give the world. Your confidence will come from knowing who you are and being comfortable with who you are. You can never be a genuine if you are an imitation. One thing I tell my students at John Robert Powers

is that you are a genuine peach. Now the girl next to you might be a genuine banana. You look at her and say, 'I want to be a banana. I don't want to be a peach anymore.' So what you make yourself into is a plastic banana. But if you were a genuine peach, which is what you were created to be, you would be a *genuine* peach. So why spend your life being an imitation?" Find out what it is you are, what is different about you, and what makes you *you*.

Factors Which To Into the Score

In addition to the verbal interaction in the judges' interview, there are other factors which to into the resulting score. The common denominator to these factors is projecting confidence and self-assurance. The very first thing judges notice about a contestant, before she even opens her mouth to introduce herself, is her appearance. She should be wearing a dress that compliments her figure, personality and skin tone, and her makeup should be appropriate and flattering.

Dressing for the Interview

The most flattering type of outfit is a simple dress, suit or contemporary combination. Jane Jaffe advises, "The proper outfit for the interview competition is an outfit that you look good in, that looks appropriate to the time of day, to the season, and to your age." Cheryl Prewitt-Salem advises that clothing worn a little loosely will give the illusion that you are thinner. Additionally, "Wearing the same color nylons and shoes can make you look taller because a single shade draws the eye up and down in one long, smooth vertical line."

This look need not be expensive. "Look into second-hand shops, estate sales and borrow from friends. What is necessary is a classic, elegant look. This elegant look, with glamorous touches, are what sets a Queen apart from a pretty girl. This look is accomplished by choice of style, fabric, texture, line, color and accessories," suggests Barbara Kelley. "See my book *What Should I Wear to Interview That Will Look Great and Not Cost My Father a Fortune* for more details."

You may wear any shoe style that complements your outfit. You should consider, however, that shoes with straps will cut that long, graceful, unbroken line you are working to create. Cheryl Prewitt-Salem recommends that you "never wear shoes that are of a lighter color than your clothing, unless you want your feet to look huge! Wear lighter-colored shoes only if you want to accent your feet." In addition, "never wear low-heeled shoes if you are short and want to seem taller. Choose shoes with a higher heel. Even a small heel, when worn with casual clothes, will make you look taller and cause you to stand up straighter." Donna Lee notes, "Shoes should always be neutral and not cause attention to the feet — after all, the face is really where the attention should be." Heeled shoes place leg muscles in a different alignment than do flat shoes. This different alignment creates a flattering leg shape.

There is no excuse for scuffs or run-down heels. If your shoes are not immaculate, your scores in grooming will be low. Depending upon the color or the shoe and its fabric, spots on most shoes can often be removed with soap and water, lighter fluid, or nail polish remover. The fact that you cannot afford another pair of expensive shoes does not excuse sloppiness. The quality of your shoes doesn't matter; you will be wearing them for only a short time. In this instance, appearance far outweighs quality.

While being original helps to set you apart from other contestants, Christy Cole recommends that "The dress should not be so outlandish that the judges remember you unfavorably." Mary Francis Flood adds, "If you are in doubt as to what to wear in any phase of competition, keep in mind that simplicity is elegance." "Dress like the job you want — that of a queen," says Barbara Kelley. "The more a contestant cares about what she is wearing, the more she cares about herself and would make a good winner. Neatness, tailoring and general good grooming is more important than actual wardrobe" notes Donna Lee. Avoid fabrics that wrinkle easily and hats, gloves or purses that can deflect the judges' attention from the contestant. Similarly, the best jewelry matches or complements the outfit with which it is worn. It is always better to under-accessorize. When in doubt, less is best.

Rules That Apply to Sitting

There are basic rules that apply to sitting. After approaching the chair, turn and step back until you feel the chair against the back of your legs. Sit down on the edge of the chair, using your leg muscles to bear your weight. Slide back halfway, sitting on the front half of the chair. Throughout the process remember to keep your back straight, avoid looking down, bending from the waist or sticking your derriere out behind you. If you will be more at ease with your back resting against the chair, do so gracefully without plopping yourself down. A body carelessly sprawled shows nothing to its best advantage. If you must smooth your skirt before sitting, do it quickly, with one hand, in a smooth motion. Sit serenely, not rigidly in the chair. A rigid pose conveys nervousness. Above all, be comfortable and maintain good posture. Avoid crossing your legs. Crossing the leg over the knee creates a very flattering distortion of the calf. You may cross your feet at the ankles. A girl with beautiful legs, who sits upright in a chair with her knees together and her ankles crossed shows her legs to their best advantage. If you must cross your legs, do so above the knee and angle your legs to one side. It is more important for you to be at ease in the interview than for your legs to be in the "correct" position. However, a nervous foot can ruin your interview and drive the judges crazy! While being interviewed, you may lean forward occasionally. If this comes naturally, it shows sincerity and alertness.

To get out of the chair, slide toward the edge of the seat. Keeping your back straight, lift with your thighs. Do not bend forward. "Don't push off with your hands or scoop up like a bird ducking for a fish in the water. Just stand straight up. Make your legs do all the work," says Cheryl Prewitt-Salem. If the chair is deep, use your knuckles gracefully to push yourself upward and forward. Do not spread your finger to use the flat side of your palm.

The Talent Competition

If you have never thought of yourself as talented, don't despair. Imagination and stage presence will carry you through. More than anything, the talent segment is a competition of creativity. Seek a cleaver way to present an interest or hobby. Over the years pageants have witnessed talents in cooking, sewing, writing, figure skating, suitcase packing, and horsemanship. In one *American Junior Miss* pageant, a contestant painted eggshells onstage, while in a *Miss California* pageant, another performed a routine that poked fun at aerobic instructors. Many contestants mistakenly feel that singing, dancing, or playing a musical instrument are the only valid talents. Lee Meriwether, *Miss America* 1954, loves to be remembered for her somber dramatic reading from "Riders to the Sea," by Irish dramatist John Millington Synge. Any talent can be successful, as long as it entertains the public.

Requirements for Talent

The absolute requirements for a talent include that it fit the pageant's guidelines — it must not involve danger, like fire batons or juggling knives, it must not involve bringing animals on stage, and it must not contain offensive material. Most pageants have a time limit for talent presentations. Generally, this is 2 minutes 50 seconds. It is always wise to plan for your presentation to take less than the allotted time. This allows you to leave the audience wanting more and provides a cushion should something effect the timing during its actual performance.

If your talent involves your own original work, such as painting or song writing, you are responsible for providing the pageant with notarized authentication that the work is your own creation. Similarly, if your pageant is televised, it is important that you clear your material for performance. This is to ensure that no copyrights are infringed upon. It is wise to have a backup talent prepared in the event that your cannot clear your original choice.

If a Mishap Occurs

Remember that the judges and audience want you to do well. They look forward to your performance and will be sympathetic if a mishap occurs. Do not become upset if you make a mistake. If a mishap should occur, Barbara Kelley advises, "Roll with the punches. Do some deep-breathing exercises. Find something humorous about the situation and laugh about it." Your best protection against mishap, however, is preparation. Visit the stage to get a sense of the place, to identify any potential hazards — such as slippery floors. One way to combat stage fright is to practice your talent in front of a mirror. This allows you to conquer the sensation of "being watched." Another way is to be so over-prepared in your presentation, that you can do it in your sleep, without conscious thought or concentration. If you find it difficult to create facial expressions, Jacque Mercer, *Miss America* 1949, suggests that you practice by reading fairy tales to children. This is just one of the helpful suggestions contained in her book, *How to Win a Beauty Contest.*

The Right Stuff

The way to reach this level of preparation is through having the right talent and having presented it before audiences so often that your body can do it on its own. To select the right talent, have someone other than family members critique your talent. Deborah Mosley won the *Miss Georgia* 1978 title with a rendition of "Summertime" from *Porgy and Bess.* After the competition, she arranged for the music director of the Columbus, Georgia public school system to help find a selection which properly demonstrated her soprano voice.

After you have found and learned the proper talent, take and make every opportunity to perform it before an audience — any audience no matter how large or small, formal or impromptu. Schools, civic meetings, churches, nursing homes, hospitals and recreation programs are just some of the possibilities for finding audiences to help you polish your stage presence.

Quality Sound

Quality sound is of utmost importance when performing. There are four types of microphones available. These are the stand mike, the wired hand mike, the wireless hand mike and the lavaliere wireless or body-pack mike. This last type straps onto your body and is small enough to fit under your talent costume. Plan on using a wired mike, unless the pageant hall has excellent audio equipment. If your talent requires a wireless mike, the hand mike usually provides more dependable sound quality than does the lavaliere. Decide which type of microphone you need by determining the movements needed to execute your talent and the limitations of the audio system at the pageant hall.

Whichever microphone you use, practice with it until you feel secure. Practice until you forget that it is there. Learn to keep the mike just an inch below your chin at all times, even when turning your head from side to side. This prevents the mike from covering your face. Also learn to pull down on full-voice notes without causing distortion. It may sound easy, but it does take practice.

Back-Up Tapes

If your talent requires accompaniment, many companies produce quality back-up performance tapes, often called Tracks. These tapes contain only the orchestration, allowing the performer to provide the vocal. Appendix E includes a list of companies which sell Tracks.

Talent Checklist and Pointers

Here is a checklist with some pointers to aid your preparation for your talent competition.

Talent Checklist:

- Song
- Sheet music
- Accompaniment
- Orchestration
- Lighting
- Props
- Microphone
- Stage Curtain (open or closed)
- Scenery
- Costumes

Talent Pointer:

- Whatever your talent may be, always go back for more lessons so you can get new pointers and more rehearsal.
- When selecting your talent, be honest with yourself about what you can and cannot do.
- When using facial expressions, exaggerate and animate them.
- Be punctual for your presentation.
- Use good manners.
- Have your talent equipment ready well before your time to entertain.

- Keep your costumes and equipment together and be neat while in the dressing rooms.
- Do not interfere with other talent onstage with either loud talk or distraction action.
- Follow all stage director's instructions.
- Be present when it is your time to compete.
- Avoid beginning your talent with your back to the audience. Try a more original opening scene.
- If you make a mistake in talent, don't lose your poise. Smile and go on from there, as quickly as possible.
- Do not thank the audience after your presentation. They thank you with their applause.
- Make a dramatic and graceful bow (or curtsy) after your presentation.
- Do not leave character until you are completely off stage.
- Remember to smile throughout your time on stage.

Summary

To summarize, talent should be fun and an enjoyable experience for all. Present yourself in the best manner possible. Have "stage presence," the ability to project your talent to the audience and completely lose yourself in your presentation. Placing your true personality in your talent is the most vital ability in your competition. Learn to command the stage with your presence and your performance.

The Swimsuit Competition

The swimsuit competition may be the hardest. Many contestants can affirm that they are exhibiting more in their swimsuits than just their legs and figures. The swimsuit competition displays the total woman — how she cares about herself as well as how she looks. A body that is physically well-conditioned reflects a woman's mental discipline. Donna Lee comments, "Swimsuit competition illustrates how much class a girl has." Standing in a swimsuit and high heels in front of strangers is hard. After this, job interviews are a cinch!

For the swimsuit competition, a girl should wear a classic maillot in a solid color. While flowers and decorations are now allowed in some pageants, a plain, solid color presents a flattering, unbroken line. The bra should provide support in the bust area. If it is unlined, sew-in bra cups can be purchased from a fabric store. Wear a suit that compliments your figure. "If it takes large breasts to make that particular suit look good, and you have a small chest, do not wear it," advises Christy Cole. "By the same token, those who are particularly big in the chest should not wear a suit that is too revealing." Judges are not impressed by a panoramic view of either your wishbone or your hip. Even if allowed, too many designs and too high a French cut are distracting to the eye. Donna Lee suggests that a good rule of thumb for a French cut swimsuit is that it should be "two inches above the thickest part of your thigh, no higher." She also recommends, "Do not wear strapless suits — your bust will sag. Small busted girls should not wear halter-strapped swimsuits."

Swimsuits should completely cover your derriere. You must be able to sit and then stand again without having the bottom ride up. If your suit keeps "creeping up on you," a product called "Firm Grip" can be found in sporting goods stores. It comes in a spray or in a tube, is colorless, will not stain and will hold your swimsuit bottom in place. Double-sided tape on your derriere will also keep your suit from riding up. The worst mistake you can make is not completely covering your derriere.

Finding the Right Suit

A modest one-piece swimsuit that meets your pageant requirements and is still sexy enough to show off your assets is not easy to find. A good designer can make a custom suit for you in the exact color and style you desire, or if you already have a good swimsuit, it can be altered at the leg or in other details. A Texas designer, Ada Duckett has invented the "supersuit" — a white maillot that has won a swimsuit award every year since 1979. In 1978, she created five of them — and they all ended up in the Top 10. *Miss America* 1972, Laurie Lea Schaefer and *Miss America* 1980, Cheryl Prewitt-Salem also realized the need for stylish and updated pageant swimsuits. Each has designed a pageant line of suits that are available to anyone who wants help. Information on all three swimsuit sources can be found in Appendix D.

Tips That Can Boost Your Confidence

While it was controversial when Susan Akin, *Miss America* 1985, admitted that she had used an adhesive to keep her swimsuit from riding up when she walked down the runway, in truth it has been done for years. In fact, it is nothing compared to other competition stratagems. Everything from padding to cosmetic surgery has been tried to perfect the swimsuit body. Some contestants wrap their bodies in cellophane to sweat off excess water weight; others minimize their waists by cinching them in with tape or use surgical tape to tape their breasts together.

There are less extreme and more beneficial tips that can aid your confidence level in the swimsuit competition. First of all, remember that this is not a sex contest. It is also very different from swimsuit modeling, so fashion show maneuvers will fall flat in a pageant. Avoid using baby oil on your body during the swimsuit competition. Oil looks greasy and will make your body look heavier. It also causes light to gleam off your body in an unnatural way. Hand or body lotion are more effective moisturizers. Prior to appearing onstage under hot lights, place a cotton ball or tissue into the cleavage of your swimsuit to absorb perspiration. If you have fair skin, a touch of blusher on your shoulders will add color. Blusher can also be used to contour your cleavage. Remember that the makeup for the swimsuit and evening gown competitions are generally glamorous. If you coordinate the color of your outfits for these two areas, the same makeup will flatter both. This is a particular advantage since there is not time to reapply makeup between stage competitions.

Jewelry is distracting during the swimsuit competition. Never wear more than simple, casual earrings, and avoid those if at all possible. If permitted, pantyhose, worn under your swimsuit, can even out skin tone and camouflage discolorations. If worn, the hose should match your skin tone so completely as to be invisible. Unfortunately, pantyhose seams can also cause a slight bulge around the waist and stomach areas. This can be minimized by cutting out the waistband and painting clear nail polish around the raw edge to help prevent runs.

The Body Condition and Posture

The body, condition and posture, are important factors in the swimsuit competition. Your posture can be improved if you exercise with small weights. Muscle tone, or lack of it, is most noticeable in this area of competition. Most judges feel that legs are the best barometer of body tone. Barbara Kelley advises, "Have your body in great shape so you'll walk proud!"

Shoes to Wear with Your Swimsuit

Never wear open-toed, open-heeled or completely flat shoes to model your swimsuit. You should also avoid wedges or shoes with wooden heels. Regular pumps with the highest possible heel in a color to match or complement your swimsuit are the safest choices. Some contestants prefer a skin-tone or nude pump to lengthen the look of the leg. Cheryl Prewitt-Salem has designed a high-heeled acrylic shoe with a "notice me, not my shoes" look. It features a completely clear heel and toe with a camel-colored leather strap that runs along the back of the heel. This shoe is available in sizes 5 to 10 and in medium and narrow widths. The shoe is not available in half-sizes. For ordering information, see Appendix D.

Focus on Your Legs

With so much focus on your legs, you should concentrate on this area when you exercise. You can do assorted leg exercises while watching television, or you can get a great workout from Cheryl Prewitt-Salem's low and high impact aerobic exercise video tapes. For more information about these tapes, see Appendix C.

The Evening Gown Competition

The evening gown competition is your opportunity to impress the judges with your elegance. You will want a gown that will make you look like a million dollars and feel enchanting. It should be made of a magic fabric. The dress must come to life under the pageant's lights. Stephanie Raye, 1988 *Miss American Petite*, selected a royal purple gown in classic lines with some gathering and bugle beading on the bodice. Stephanie remembers, "I wanted to shine over it [her gown]. I wanted the judges to notice me — not the dress."

Choosing a Pageant Gown

Pageant gown styles change from pageant season to pageant season. Years ago, full-skirted chiffon styles were popular. Today, a contestant wearing too many ruffles is making a mistake. The recent trend, in fact, has been to more glamorous gowns. Keep up with the trends in evening gowns by attending pageants or watching them on television.

For your own gown, look for something different — but not too different. Avoid the passe relics of years gone by, including hoop skirts, pageant capes, gloves and long chiffon scarves floating from around the neck. Avoid strapless gowns because they distort the bust. Similarly, reject very tight, backless or very low cut gowns which call attention to a chubby back. Balance the look of a one-shouldered gown by wearing your hair on the side of your bare shoulder. If you are having a one-shouldered gown made, have the shoulder going in the same direction as the winner's banner. The most successful contestants are wearing gowns that don't hinder their movement. Simplicity is best; gowns should not be fussy. The current trend is to classic, straight, form fitting gowns which impart height and sophistication, but wearing this style requires a good figure. When you begin to see many contestants in a particular style, it is time for you to find a different one.

The gown you choose must be appropriate for your age. A teen trying to look like an adult is just as embarrassing as an adult trying to look like a teen. There is no place for sexy gowns in a teen pageant. At the same time, avoid the "country fair" styles. Teens should look and dress like teens and not try to look older. Strive for the "wholesome, all-American, girl-next-door" look that will cause the judges to look at you and say, "There's a pretty girl." You don't want them to think, "Wow, there goes a beauty queen." A young girl who projects sex appeal *is* handicapped in a teen pageant.

Sparkle

If your evening gown has a lot of sparkle, little jewelry needs to be worn. Avoid wearing heavy rhinestone necklaces. If you feel you need more sparkle, add a stream of rhinestones edge of the bodice. Short contestants, especially, should avoid having bands of color break up the line of their gowns. Particularly, avoid having the bodice and skirt of different colors. Watches, rings and bracelets also break the visual line and distract the eye. They should not be worn with competition outfits.

Cost

Some girls spend a lot of money on their gowns while others spend what they can. An attractive, long, drop-dead evening gown that will show up well on stage usually means a gown with sequins or rhinestones. It is difficult to find one of these for less than $200, but many girls rent their gowns. With patience, you can find a gown perfect for your pageant at a reasonable price. Purchasing a gown and adding rhinestones is a common practice among pageant contestants. One contestant bought a simple evening gown for $10 at a rummage sale and added rhinestones in a swirling pattern encircling the gown at the hips. She then cut off the original straps and added rhinestone straps. Needless to say, the gown looked beautiful!

Grooming and Taste

Pageant coach Mary Francis Flood stresses grooming and good taste over spending lots of money. Donna Lee notes, "Clothes play an important part in a girl winning, but it's what's in the clothes that counts. When judging, I look at what the girl does for the gown, not what the gown does for the girl. No contest should ever be a clothing competition." When Michelle Royer won the *Miss USA* title in 1987, one state director protested at the pageant in Albuquerque, "We cannot afford a $40,000 gown like *Miss Texas*. Texas directors Richard Guy and Rex Holt spent a total of $350 on the gown, saying that "Velvet is cheap." Besides, money does not make the gown, the women wearing it does. *Miss Denton* Lesly Braun competed in the *Miss Texas* pageant, wearing the gown Phyllis George wore for the talent competition in the *Miss America* pageant. Unfortunately, even though she had borrowed *Miss America's* gown, Lesly did not become *Miss Texas*.

When searching for the perfect gown, look for one that compliments your figure as well as your skin tone. You have to wear it, it can't wear you. Christy Cole warns, "You should not wear something so outlandish that it makes you look silly. The judges will remember, but it won't be favorable." If you plan to enter many pageants, it may be worth the investment to have a designer or seamstress make gowns especially for you. Unless you are an excellent seamstress, hire a professional. Evening gowns worn in competition should never look homemade.

A Nightmare is Finding Another Contestant Wearing Your Gown

One potential nightmare is finding another contestant wearing a gown that is identical to yours. According to *The Beauty Pageant Manual*, although this is disappointing and embarrassing, it does not affect the scoring and makes no difference to the judges. In fact, except for contestants such as San Diego's *Fairest of the Fair* pageant in which all contestants compete in identical gowns, it is rare for two girls to have chosen identical gowns. If this should happen to you, however, don't worry. Donna Lee suggests that wearing the same gown can actually work to your advantage. "The girl appearing in the gown that looks the best will undoubtedly get the higher score." When asked his opinion of contestants competing in identical gowns, Ted Marshall, editor of the *Pageant Review*, stated, "Now, this would be a true competition! They would have to be judged better due to their individual efforts or God-given talents or features." Jane Jaffe remembers that her daughter, Lisa, competed twice in contests in which another contestant was wearing a gown which was identical to hers. Jane did not think that this had affected the outcome. "The judges are certainly not going to take off points for that. It's not going to affect them in any way, other than making one feel that someone else stole her thunder. What you have to figure is we're two different people, and we wear it two different ways."

Shoes

The best shoe for evening gown competition is a classic pump that matches or complements your gown. Never wear open-toed, open-heeled, or completely flat shoes in the evening gown competition. Sandals draw attention to the feet — away from the gown and the contestant in it. Furthermore, sandal straps tend to break at the most inconvenient moments. The right shoe need not be expensive. Simple pumps are the least expensive shoes. If you prefer dressier evening shoes, add your own rhinestones in a design you like, and save on the expense. Cheryl Prewitt-Salem competed for the *Miss Mississippi* title wearing a pair of shoes that were spray-painted red crimson and doused with red glitter. Up close, they reminded Cheryl of a failed arts-and-crafts project, but from a distance they were beautiful. This technique can be used to make dazzling evening shoes or talent competition shoes (which is what Cheryl actually did). Satin shoes take dye better than other fabric shoes and are dressier, but according to *The Beauty Pageant Manual*, dyed pumps often fade onto hosiery around the edges of the shoe — even after weeks of drying time. To protect from this ruining your look, bring several pairs of nylons.

New shoes should be broken in before the pageant. Avoid sore feet at pageant events by wearing shoes around the house until they are comfortable. If they are tight, you can loosen them up by wearing them with socks. You can also add heel grips, toe pads, and full length cushion soles, if your shoes are uncomfortable. If your shoe soles are too slippery, you can make them rougher by taking the new shoe outdoors and rubbing the soles across concrete. You can also create rougher surface by putting masking tape over the soles or abrading the surface of the sole with an emery board. Slippery soles should be corrected as unattended, since they could cause you to slip on the runway.

Onstage

Once you have created the perfect evening gown competition ensemble, you must perfect the way you will present it onstage. You may think that your walk is graceful, but sometimes we are not able to do an accurate self-evaluation. To be certain, it would be to your advantage to tape your stance and walk. If you do not own a video camera, many stores will rent them by the day. When you look at a tape of yourself, you will be able to see if you are doing anything that is less than flattering. If a video tape is just not possible, ask a friend who is familiar with pageant modeling or a teacher who seems poised and self-confident to evaluate you and provide helpful suggestions.

If you have balance problems when turning, you probably have either neglected to shift your weight between turns, thus starting with the wrong foot, i.e. back foot first, or you have taken one step too many and turned in the wrong way. Practice remembering which foot must end in front to turn in the correct direction. It will be helpful to know how to turn on either side — just in case you end up on the wrong foot.

If you find you are stepping on your gown, it is because you are titling your body forward. This can be due to heels that are too high or just not knowing how to walk properly in high heels. Practice walking in front of a mirror with a book on your head. When you no longer drop your book, you have corrected your tilt.

Contestants should carry themselves with pride, walking with poise, elegance and grace, like a Queen. Your walk should be smooth, deliberate and purposeful, commanding attention. It should not be too bouncy or too peppy. At the same time, it should not be too stiff. A rigid walk makes you look ill at ease. Many times a girl wins a pageant by having learned how to walk, talk, sit, and appear self-confident. You can make the most striking and winning impression on the judges and the audience by having learned to walk elegantly.

Walk on the balls of your feet — not on your heels or on your toes. Place one foot slightly in front of the other. Lift the spine up tall, projecting height, lean slightly forward and feel the ball of your foot as you walk. Look natural and don't hurry. The correct walk can be learned, but it cannot be faked. The secret to perfect poise is that it never looks studied.

Walk smoothly with movement only from your hips down. Keep your upper body from moving and your hips and derriere from swaying or wiggling. Your feet should be pointed straight ahead, walking so that you lead and glide with the balls of your feet. Do not tiptoe. Your head should not bob when you walk. Your arms should swing naturally, neither exaggerating the motion nor stifling it. Only your arms should move, not your shoulders. Your thighs should slightly brush each other while you walk.

When it is your turn to be presented onstage, stand with both feet together, facing the audience. Angle one foot in back to the 10:00 or 2:00 position, depending on which foot is in back. The front foot should face forward at the 12:00 position. Your weight should be centered on your back foot, but evenly distributed from side to side. Your tummy is sucked in, and your derriere is tucked under. Both knees are slightly bent, but not locked. In fact, your knees should never be locked because a forgotten, locked knee can throw off your balance. Do not throw one hip out to the side. In fact, the stance just described will automatically tilt the hips slightly, deflecting the straight-on view which would make you look wider.

Smile and Eye Contact

When onstage, always smile and maintain good eye contact with the judges. Look each judge in the eye, giving them your best smile. "You have the rest of your lives to look at your friends and relatives that might be in the audience. It is the judges who hold your future in their hands at this moment," advises Christy Cole. You can look briefly at all areas of the audience, but, she continues, "Absolutely no winking and no sexy looks should accompany your smile!" She recommends that you prepare for this situation. "Contestants should also look at themselves in the mirror, stretching their chin out and peek underneath at their neck. Not a very pleasant sight is it? That is what the judges see when you look out into the audience and not directly at them!"

Before you begin your walk down the runway, pause. Wait for the attention of the audience, then proceed with one foot directly in front of the other. DO NOT RUSH! The excitement of the event will make you tend to speed up, so concentrate on walking slowly. If you can count a cadence in your head and walk to it, you can reduce the tendency to race. Rushing betrays nerves and reduces the time the judges have to evaluate you. When you come down a runway, your head should move from side to side, sweeping the audience and acknowledging the judges. When you cross the front of the stage, angle your shoulders slightly toward the audience and look in that direction. Before going off stage pause again for one last look. Remember to walk and turn slowly, and above all, SMILE! Your smile should remain on your face until you are completely offstage and out of sight. If you should happen to walk offstage in the wrong direction, continue walking because it will be more noticeable if you correct it. If you should happen to trip or fall onstage, — at any time, — immediately resume your position without losing either poise or composure.

Chapter 3

APPEARANCE: GROOMING TECHNIQUES

Being a beauty queen is more than wearing a crown and a queens wardrobe, makeup and hairstyle. When a titleholder flashes that royal smile, she reveals well tended teeth. When her plane is late and the weather is atrocious and her luggage is lost and the interviewer asks a rude question, a queen knows how to suppress her immediate reaction, reduce stress, take a deep breath and remain the embodiment of graciousness and poise. These are traits that have to be developed and maintained before the pageant. The judges are seeking a titleholder who already possesses these abilities. Your preparation for pageant competition should include time on the "internals."

Good Grooming

Good grooming is one universal pageant requirement. It is imperative in every pageant and in every area of competition, as well as every time contestants are in public view. Looking your best gives you confidence and a sense of control. Confidence enables you to relax and be more open and friendly. This, in turn, encourages others to act warmly toward you. Good grooming habits set off a "spiral of success." Barbara Kelley says, "I'm astounded by chipped polish, runs in stockings, unpressed dresses and black bras under light colored tops. I can't believe my eyes!" Donna Lee notes, "Good grooming is always an asset. I believe if a girl takes care of herself, she will do the title justice. I even pay attention to nails and to scuff marks on shoes. I detest runs in hose and gaudy jewelry only detracts from the contestant." Successful pageant contestants have come to realize that physical appearance and good grooming are much more than a matter of simple vanity. Looks are a form of self-expression that influence how others see you, as well as how you see yourself.

Express Your Good Taste

Send the message that you are a person who cares enough about herself to let her warmth, competence, and zest for life show. Express your good taste in your grooming and wardrobe choices. Stay away from extremely faddish styles. Most judges find tight-fitting evening gowns less flattering than gowns with fullness in the skirt — especially on young women. Extremely low cut dresses are always considered to be an example of bad taste. They should be avoided.

Tanning

A light golden color imparts a "healthy glow," but avoid getting a dark tan. Beauty pageant are *not* tanning contests. Additionally, dark tanned faces do not take makeup well and may not look natural. If you insist on tanning, do not develop tan lines. Furthermore, sunbathe during the less hazardous hours, either before 10 a.m. or after 3 p.m. Always wear a sunscreen with a rating of at least 15 to minimize your exposure to cancer causing ultraviolet radiation. Avoid tanning salons altogether. They cause a host of problems, including corneal burns, cataracts, damaged blood vessels, and a weakened immune system, not to mention prematurely wrinkled skin. Tanning salons are still unlicensed and unregulated in all but three U.S. states and often times owners don't warn customers of health risks. If you insist on a high-tech tan, take these precautions:

1. Always wear goggles. Just closing your eyes won't protect you from ultraviolet radiation.
2. Use only booths equipped with automatic timers.
3. Do not make pseudo-sunning (or real sunning) sessions a habit.

Color Analysis

Know your best and worst colors — which ones do well in competition, which are the most common and should thus be avoided. Some colors produce predictable reactions in people. The basic rule of color is that dark colors slim and light colors enlarge. Knowing the psychology of color will help. For example, interviewing someone in red at the end of a long hard day can be irritating; blue is relaxing, and white is refreshing. Karen Kemple advises, "Contestants should not choose colors that most people dislike (shades of brown, orange, etc.) unless worn in small amounts." Outfits in solid colors are sophisticated, eye-catching and flattering.

Many girls do not know their best colors. If you can afford it, have your makeup colors analyzed by a professional color analyst and learn some of their techniques. If you cannot afford to see a professional, expert advice can be found in Carole Jackson's book *Color Me Beautiful*. Karen Kemple seconds, "In competition, you must know and wear your best colors from an objective viewpoint, rather than your own personal favorites." If you cannot afford to see a professional makeup consultant or color analyst, consult Jackson's book *Color Me Beautiful Makeup Book*. It is vital for you to know which makeup colors are right for your skin tone. You also need to consider the effect that a color has on your hair. If a color looks great with your skin tone and in the fabric but makes your hair look lifeless because there is not enough contrast, your hair will not look good, no matter what you do with it.

Colors

White is the most common color in pageantry. It also has the best winning record. It is a safe color. In the 1988 *Miss South Carolina USA* pageant, eleven out of twelve finalists wore white evening gowns. However, "Girls with yellowish-colored teeth should avoid wearing white, especially near their face," says color consultant Thelma Pratt. "It would only make their teeth look darker." Royal blue is a striking color and shows up well onstage. Red is also popular in pageants, although it can look gaudy in the wrong fabric and style. Remember that the effect of a color will depend entirely on the fabric. Colors appear stronger in sequined fabric while they appear lighter in sheerer fabric. Emerald is often worn by girls with winter complexions. Fuchsia is another good stage color and can be stunning if it suits your hair and skin. Turquoise is also popular and luckily, it is flattering to everyone. Recently, black gowns have gained in popularity in competitions, but remember that black should not be worn near the face. In the 1988 *Miss USA* pageant, three of the ten semifinalists wore black gowns. The ultimate winner, Courtney Gibbs, *Miss Texas USA*, was one of them.

Positive Ways to Stand Out

Work to avoid getting "lost in the crowd." Knowing positive ways to stand out is a competitive edge. There are many ways you can differentiate yourself from the other contestants. During competition, contestants who have a gimmick, such as a one-color wardrobe or a one-shouldered gown and swimsuit, can make it easier for the judges to remember them. Whenever you have a choice of what to wear, pick something that will be memorable. Choose a dress in a bright solid color rather than a skirt and blouse. Another gimmick might be matching competition outfits to your eye color or wearing the same hairstyle for all areas of competition (rather than leaving it down for the swimsuit and up for the evening gown). Karen Kemple recalls, "Contestants have been known to wear an obvious big piece of jewelry on their interview outfit, knowing it will draw the judges' attention. When a judge comments on the jewelry, she can give a small history about it, guiding them into an area she is in control of."

Jewelry

Dressy earrings can be worn with the evening gown. These can range from simple pearls or diamonds to larger styles. The fact to remember is that the size earring you choose should be appropriate for the size and shape of your features. If you have a short neck, do not wear long, dangling earrings; small features require smaller earrings. Karen Kemple suggests that earrings can also be used to balance or correct ones face shape. While a necklace is generally permitted, Barbara Kelley suggests that you stick with earrings alone — "no necklaces or bracelets."

Pageant Makeup

Pageant makeup should be matte, never frosted. Matte makeup can be applied more heavily than frosted, without looking artificial. Additionally, frosted makeup brings out skin imperfections.

Cover all scars, birthmarks, veins, and other imperfections with makeup. Avoid shine by dusting your face with a face powder. Tinted powder will turn orange after long hours on the face and look unnatural when retouched. Translucent powder, on the other hand, allows you to touch up without looking patched up. Country music star Barbara Mandrell suggests using baby powder because it is even more translucent than face powder. Whichever you use, apply the powder liberally to avoid shine, keep a matte look and set makeup to avoid smudges. Pick up the excess by rolling a cotton ball around your entire face as a final step.

Tips

Waterproof products work very well for some women, holding up better during times of stress. Many girls cry under stress, so waterproof mascara is a real boon. Max Factor recently created "No Color Mascara," a crystal clear mascara that avoids the problem-causing heavy colorants of traditional mascara. Its clear formula is hypo-allergenic and is perfect for girls who want longer, darker lashes without sacrificing natural eyes.

Choose a lip color shade that blends with or complements your cheek color. Avoid colors that make your teeth appear yellowish. Before applying your lip color, outline your lips with a lip liner pencil in a shade complementary to your lipstick. Do not use a lip liner color that contrasts with your lipstick. Lip lining is an art that it is wise to master. It can be used to slightly alter the shape of ones lips, or it can be applied over the entire lip surface, before the lipstick is applied. This latter technique will set the lipstick and help it last for hours. Other techniques which will help your lip color last include using a dry formula, matte lipstick, powdering between coats, and avoiding gloss. "If you do use it," advises Karen Kemple of lip gloss, "apply it only in the center of your lips. This will highlight the center without making your lipstick bleed."

"Cheek color should be applied in deeper shades (for stage)," says Karen Kemple, "to define cheekbones and should be blended to avoid a masked look." Contour makeup may be powder, liquid base, or stick. It is about two shades darker than the foundation makeup and can be used for stage, but only if you know how to apply it correctly. Learning to contour your face effectively is the most difficult aspect of makeup artistry.

Never apply makeup under fluorescent lights because it distorts the true colors. Also, white and pastel colors reflect light onto the face. When purchasing makeup, Karen Kemple advises that you wear a blouse that matches the color of the gown you will be wearing. Sample the makeup and step outside into the sunlight to see the true color.

Makeup Intensity

Perfect the makeup that you will use for each area of competition. In all phases of competition, cosmetic choices should be soft and natural. Stay away from harsh tones and avoid pale lipsticks. The heavy use of makeup is usually unflattering — it makes the judges ask "What is she trying to hide?" Even onstage, with bright lights, makeup should be natural. Interview makeup should be natural but polished. It should not be noticeable. A line where the makeup begins and ends can be erased with a sponge. Know the setting of your interview ahead of time so that you can adjust the intensity of your palette for the brightness of the lighting. As mentioned above, fluorescent lighting can dull and distort makeup colors. Makeup for the evening gown competition should be very glamorous. However, it should enhance your appearance rather than being the focal point. It should be well defined, so that you can be seen from a distance. This does not mean that the actual application should be heavier, only that the colors should be more intense. Eye makeup should be darker during the evening gown competition. If you use false eyelashes to supplement your own, the lashes should be individually applied, followed by a coat of mascara to blend the artificial lashes with your own.

Talent makeup is even more intensified than that of the swimsuit or evening gown competitions. Though it looks heavy close up, it will be just right from the audience's point of view. Nevertheless, contestants should be careful not to go overboard, appearing "made-up." Choose matte makeup, not frosted, and stay away from trendy gimmicks like adding glitter to the corner of your eyes. The judges want elegance, not flashiness.

Two factors should be considered in determining the intensity of your makeup. These are the lighting and the distance to the audience. By this criteria, your makeup intensity should differ when you are one-on-one, onstage, or on television.

You will need to get used to applying and wearing the more intense makeup that will keep you from fading out onstage. You can experiment and have free makeup applications in department stores by professional artists. Before purchasing cosmetics, ask for various sample with which to experiment at home. You will need to learn to apply your own makeup properly and quickly — in five minutes! While some pageants provide makeup artists to assist their contestants, you should know how to do your own in the event of an emergency.

Camouflage

There are many features you can learn to enhance and minimize by experimenting with makeup. If you have a round face, you can thin it out by shading your blush beneath the cheekbone and above the jaw. Karen Kemple recommends, "You can make your lips appear fuller by painting a lighter shade (highlight) in the center and by painting just beyond the borders." If you have extremely blond eyebrows, you can darken them with an eyebrow pencil or brush on a coat of dark mascara. Mascara not only helps define the eyebrow, it helps keep eyebrow hairs in place. Darker eyebrows are visible from a greater distance, adding dimension to your forehead.

Dazzling Clear Skin

Dazzling clear skin is essential to entering a pageant. According to a 1985 *Seventeen* magazine skin care survey, 48% of American teenage girls had had blackheads in the month before the survey. Only 26% have normal skin. These figures confirm that many girls have problem skin. If you're not one of the lucky 26%, consider visiting a well-established, licensed aesthetician to help clean your skin. An aesthetician can give you acne treatments, minimize the appearance of pockmarks, small scars and other minor skin faults, making your skin smoother than you thought possible. Aestheticians are listed in the yellow pages under Facial-Skin Care.

If you have scars from earlier skin problems, do not be concerned. You can camouflage these marks with a coverstick or foundation.

A newly introduced product, *Dermablend*, aids in covering scars. It comes in a variety of shades and is available in most department stores.

Skin Types

Professional skin treatment only supplements the regular care you give your complexion at home. No matter how much makeup you use, if your skin is in bad condition, it will show. A flawless complexion starts with good habits. It is much easier to choose a proper skin care regimen if you know your skin type. The guide below will help you determine which type most nearly matches your own.

Dry. Does your skin feel taut most of the time? Or itchy? These are signs of dry skin.

Oily. Try this simple test if you think your skin may be oily: Before washing or showering, cut a small strip from a brown paper bag and *gently* rub it against your forehead several times. If the paper shows visible traces of oil, your skin may be oilier than normal.

Part Oily/Part Dry. You have combination skin if your forehead, nose and chin — the T-zone — are oily but your cheeks aren't.

Normal. Your skin is considered normal if it is neither excessively dry nor oily, even in particular areas.

Sensitive. If your skin is temperamental, your face tends to break out in red blotches at the least provocation — say the touch of perfume in lotions and soaps.

Skin Care

Religiously practice a cleansing and conditioning routine that is appropriate for your skin type, and periodically treat your face to an even deeper cleansing of cosmetic build-up and daily grime. Give your face a sauna by steaming it. An inexpensive way to do this is with the steam of boiling water. Place water in a large pot and bring it to a boil on the stove. After the water boils, turn off the stove. With your hair pinned back or in a shower cap, position your face over the pot of steaming water with a towel over your head, making sure the steam does not escape. Stay in this position for 4 to 5 minutes, slowly turning your head from side-to-side, exposing all areas of your face. Never keep your face in one position. You will find it refreshing to remove your face from the steam from time-to-time, and inhale several deep breaths before returning to the steam. Steam can burn, so don't put your face too close to the steam and remember to keep your eyes closed. After the facial sauna, rinse your face with lukewarm water and blot your skin dry with a towel. Then apply a toner and your favorite moisturizing lotion. Avoid going out in cold weather immediately after your facial sauna.

If you prefer a simpler way to give your face a sauna, purchase *EpiSauna*, the smallest portable facial sauna on the market today. Completely portable, it folds and stands only 3 1/2" high. It uses ordinary tap water and provides voltage conversion for use anywhere in the world. With its slender styling, unique fold-down hood and travel adapter, *EpiSauna* is ready to provide all the benefits of a professional facial sauna treatment at home or on the go. *EpiSauna's* beautifying mist relaxes facial muscles and leaves the skin feeling and looking healthier and more radiant. *EpiSauna* can be purchased in most major department stores. For further information, call 1-800-238-2200.

Relaxed facial muscles make the skin feel and look healthier and more radiant. A pillow that is especially designed to eliminate pressure on the skin is a real boon. It not only helps prevent wrinkles, it may soften or erase those that have already formed. Such a pillow actually exists ad is available now. Pillow Nouveau was designed by Victoria Hall after she noticed morning sleep marks on her own face. Tested and widely endorsed, the Pillow Nouveau has been featured in articles in *Health*, *Cosmopolitan*, and *Beauty Digest*. The pillow comes with a designer slipcover, but satin slipcovers are also available at additional cost. To order your pillow, call 1-800-456-7500, extension 1500.

Overcoming Handicaps

Do not let scars deter you from competing in pageants. In her book, *A Bright Shining Place*, Cheryl Prewitt-Salem tells of many obstacles, both large and small. When she was 11 years old, Cheryl was involved in a tragic automobile accident. Her leg was severely injured, resulting in crippling disfigurement — one leg was shorter than the other. Her face was lacerated by the broken windshield. It required more than 100 stitches and left unsightly scars. Crippled and scarred, she hardly seemed a future *Miss America*. Determined to improve her appearance, Cheryl found that vitamin E oil and cocoa butter helped to minimize her scars. Additionally, Cheryl says, "The less you touch facial marks, the better off you will be. That is another reason why a sponge is better than your fingertips for applying makeup. Many times your fingers will make a scar red from touching it. Makeup will not adhere to some scars when applied by the fingers, so use that sponge!"

If you have troubled skin, consult a dermatologist as soon as possible. You may need medication or specific advice to help solve your skin problems. Never try new products right before a pageant. They may cause an allergic reaction. Experiment with new products at least two months before your pageant. People with acne-prone skin should avoid using products, including cosmetics, that contain isopropyl myristate, isopropyl neopentnoate, cetyl oleate, octyl stearate, octyl palitate, isocetyl stearate, myristyl myristate, and/or PPG 2 myristyl propionate.

On the other hand, vitamins A and K help fight bacteria and are often recommended for acne-prone skin. It is important that you note that vitamin A is highly toxic in large amounts, the proper dosage is essential to derive any benefits.

You can avoid bacteria buildup by only applying makeup to a clean face, using clean implements. Covering dirty skin with makeup only promotes blemishes. Cheryl Prewitt-Salem admonishes, "Never sleep with your makeup on; it's damaging to your face and skin. You may say, 'But I just do it now and then; I don't always have time to wash it all off.' Love your face and your skin. Do them — and yourself — a favor. No matter how tired you are, never go to bed without carefully removing your makeup."

Also, do not share your makeup with anyone. Bacteria starts growing in makeup the first time you use it. Your makeup may not affect you, but it may affect another. During the *Miss America* pageant, Marilyn Van Derbur borrowed eyeshadow from another

contestant. During the night Marilyn had to call an eye doctor.
Luckily, in spite of the trauma, Marilyn went on to become *Miss America* 1958.

Hair Styles

Pageant competition hair styles change with the times. Today, contestants should avoid extremely long hair, keeping it off the face. Too much hair on your face can hide your features. Additionally, according to Barbara Kelley, keeping your hair away from your face will help you avoid unflattering shadows from the stage lighting.

Most national contestant wear shoulder-length hair. Hair much longer than shoulder length does not flatter everyone. It projects a high school homecoming look, rather than a national beauty queen one. Additionally, long straight hair isn't as manageable, versatile, or neat-looking as it should be. At the same time, extremely short hair is similarly restrictive when it comes to varying looks. Jackie Mayer, *Miss America* 1963, was the only *Miss America* to ever wear extremely long hair. Her hair, which she wore wrapped around her head like a coronet, was reported to be 52 inches long. If you have good facial bone structure, wearing your hair "up" during the evening gown presentation can be very flattering. In any event, it is best to comb your hair fuller than you usually do — it will probably droop under hot lights. The *Miss America* hairstyle is created by teasing the hair straight out and combing it smoothly into shape, coating the resulting style with hair spray. *The Beauty Pageant Manual* contains some excellent tips on how you can use hairspray.

Select a hairstyle that is complimentary to your age and personality. Natural, soft-looking styles are the most attractive. Also, choose a style that you can easily maintain yourself. Hairdressers and stylists are not always available at pageants. Even if they happen to be available, *The Beauty Pageant Manual* warns that a stylist may fix your hair in an "extreme" style that will serve as a trademark for the designer, with little thought about what it will do for the contestant.

Your hair accentuates your features, so it is important that it emphasizes the right ones. Make sure your hair is trimmed to an even length and that split ends have been removed. Hair should be in excellent condition. This is indicated by its healthy shine. There are many ways to add shine, highlights or color to less than sparkling hair. If your hair absorbs light, rather than reflecting it, consider lightening or darkening it, so it will show up better.

Experiment Well In Advance

If you decide to try a new look, experiment well in advance to find the style and stylist who is right for you. Trying out a new color, style, permanent or stylist within months of a pageant can be very risky. Experimenting early gives you time to adjust to any changes. Plan ahead to work with someone who is familiar with pageant styles. Working early gives you time to find the style and stylist who are right for you. Richard Guy and Rex Holt suggested that Christy Fichtner wear her hair in a French twist to accent her face, making her look less like Christie Brinkley. It took months, but eventually she did get comfortable with this title-winning hairstyle.

Facial Shapes

Before you decide which hairstyle is the most flattering to your facial features, you must be aware of your facial shape. These include round, square jawed, long and narrow, high foreheaded, low foreheaded, perfect oval and narrow or pointed chin. Beauty books can help you determine what shape is yours, if you do not already know. A titleholder's hairstyle should complement her crown. Once you know what type of crown your pageant uses, you can be prepared by planning your hairstyle accordingly.

Your Smile

You probably have never thought of your dentist as a beauty consultant, but he or she is indispensable to an attractive smile. Clean, pink gums that hug a full set of white, even, stain-free teeth make a winning smile. Professional cleaning reaches places you can't, removing plaque and stains that develop no matter how conscientiously you clean your mouth. If your teeth are uneven or crooked, orthodontia can straighten them. Contestants should smile even if they wear braces. Braces are not a factor in pageant judging. Kelli Lee was crowned *Miss South Texas Teen* only days after having braces placed on her teeth. Cheryl Prewitt-Salem reflects, "The point is that most people are not as conscious of your defects as you are. Most of the time, people are not looking at your teeth nearly as much as they are looking for a smile from you. They're looking for your heart, your happiness, what is deep down inside you. It's not your face itself that's most important, it's what's coming from your face that they care about. A caring smile is always beautiful. All the world would like to receive a smile from you."

In her book *How to Win a Beauty Contest,* Jacque Mercer, *Miss America* 1949, suggests practicing your smile on someone or something that won't smile back — like lampposts and mailboxes. Kelli Lee recommends that you "work more at becoming comfortable, liking yourself and what you do, then the smile is natural." However you prepare, when onstage, the results of that preparation will be on display! Some directors tell their contestants to rub Vaseline on their teeth to facilitate hours of smiling. I, personally, don't advise this because, for most people, it just makes a mess. If you do choose to use Vaseline, place a tiny amount on the teeth. This is all that is needed to add extra brilliance under lights. If you use too much, your teeth will look greasy.

Between visits to your dentist, you have to maintain the good work he or she has done on your smile. A toothbrush and dental floss are excellent for controlling plaque, but adding baking soda, hydrogen peroxide and a dental irrigator, like WaterPik, to your antiplaque kit can keep your smile in beautiful condition. Baking soda cleans and whitens teeth and hydrogen peroxide helps to oxygenate gum pockets, stifling the growth of bacteria. Use equal parts of baking soda and hydrogen peroxide. Massage the paste into your gum line, then floss and brush. Finish with a rinse of fresh water.

Hands, Nails, and Elbows

Well-tended hands and well-groomed nails make a significant contribution to a polished, "pulled-together" look. Not only that, the condition of your hands and nails can be one of the biggest clues to how well you care for yourself. Hands should be smooth and soft. Moisturize your hands daily to avoid dryness. Get rid of dead skin cells by exfoliating your skin on a weekly basis. Exfoliation is the mild abrasion or buffing of your skin to speed up the natural shedding of surface skin cells. It has two major benefits. It deep cleans pores, and it makes the skin look fresher. Cleansing grains, an exfoliation lotion, a loofa sponge, or other skin peeler will help this weekly task. After the treatment, apply lotion or cream to the newly exposed skin. If you have dry skin, exfoliate once every other week or twice a month. You can also deep condition your hands while you sleep by slathering them with lots of cream then wearing cotton gloves.

Most pageant competitors have medium to long nails, although short nails are acceptable if they are neatly manicured. Very long nails do not flatter anyone. Remember that the longer you wear your nails, the greater the chance that you will break one of them. If you do break a nail, cut the others to the same length. If you should happen to break an artificial nail, most nail salons can do an emergency repair on relatively short notice.

Your nail color should match or complement your lipstick color. If your wardrobe colors dictate changing polish, you should choose a neutral color that will go with everything. You will not have time to change polish during the hectic pageant schedule. To avoid calling attention to your hands, you can select a clear or beige toned polish. If your nails are well tended and buffed, you do not need to wear polish at all. You should never appear with chipped nail polish. If you have problem nails, use a nail hardener with filaments. Make yellowed nails brighter-looking by using a white pencil under your tips and by foregoing nail polish until the pageant.

A pedicure is necessary if you plan to wear open-toed shoes or sandals. You may be skeptical as to whether or not a judge will bother to notice your toes. Judges have very trained, critical eyes and a talent for scanning you from head to toe, summing you up instantly. They may think, "Hmm, something is missing; she looks unfinished."

We tend to forget our elbows because they are not in eye-range, but soft elbows can always enhance your overall appearance. Start your elbow grooming process by placing a warm, wet washcloth on your elbows. Then, take an exfoliating agent (the same one you use on your hand) to remove the dead skin from this area. Next, rub half a lemon over the entire elbow to even out the skin tone. Finally, apply cream to ensure softness.

Hair Removal

The standard for pageant competition is a look as smooth as silk. There are many methods, ranging from temporary to permanent, for the removal of the body hair which detracts from this look. These methods include:

Shaving The most popular manner of removing hair is shaving with a razor. Soft, pliable hair is easier to remove, so never shave dry. Hair can soak up as much as one-third of its own weight in water, and shaving cream or soft soap helps soften the hair and lubricate the skin. Shave with long, even upward strokes, being particularly careful around the ankle bones and in the delicate, behind-the-knee area. DO NOT use shaving cream, soap or water when you are using an electric shaver. Water + electricity = electrocution.

Depilatories Chemical depilatories contain alkaline compounds that break down the structure of the hair, causing it to detach from the skin. Anything strong enough to dissolve hair, however, can also sting or burn the skin. Consequently, it is not advisable to use these products on facial hair. Also, teenagers and people with sensitive skin, should avoid depilatories.

Waxing Waxing is usually performed in salons and can be expensive, but home hair wax preparations are available. As with all preparations that you put on your skin, you should notice the ingredients and follow the directions carefully to avoid irritating your skin. Before you have a wax treatment, you must abstain from shaving the area in question for two weeks — or until you have a good enough growth for the technique to work effectively.

Bleaching Bleaching camouflages. It strips hair of its pigment, making it less visible. Because it lightens hair, bleaching works best on fair-haired, fair-skinned people. Facial hair and hair on the forearms are ideal targets for bleaching. Bleaching creams can be found in most drug or grocery stores. Be aware, however, that bleaching may leave permanent light patches on the skin.

Electrolysis Electrolysis is a procedure which permanently removes hair. A fine needle is inserted into the hair follicle, and a mild electrical charge kills each hair at the root. The dead hairs are then lifted out. If you intend to use electrolysis, find a competent, well-trained professional. Too much current can scar the skin, so don't try a home kit. For names of well-trained electrologists in your area, send your request, with a self-addressed, stamped envelope, to The International Guild of Professional Electrologists, Medical Center, 3209 Premier Drive, Suite 124, Plano, TX 75075.

Tweezing Plucking with tweezers is the most common procedure used to shape eyebrows. With tweezing, regrowth may occur in two to eight weeks. As with any other technique, there are certain precautions to follow. Use clean tweezers and watch the procedure in a magnifying mirror. Never pluck your brows further inward than the corner of your eyes; never tweeze stray hairs above the brows, and never pull a hair from a mole without first consulting a dermatologist. These, like the small hairs on the surface of the nostrils, are best cut or clipped.

Epilady Epilady, the newest method of hair removal, looks like an electric razor. It isn't. Epilady's patented coils rotate to grasp hair, removing it at the root. This achieves long lasting results similar to those of waxing. To use Epilady: Hair should be approximately 1/16" long. Wash the skin, massaging with a loofa to remove dead skin cells and raise the hair up; dry your skin, then go over the area with the Epilady, using circular motions. Regrowth takes an average of three weeks. Tests show that after using Epilady for one year, women reported that they could "epilite" both legs in approximately 15 minutes, that their hair was softer and finer, and that they would recommend Epilady to a friend. Epilady is recommended only for use on the legs and forearms. Women who do experience discomfort when first using Epilady report that the sensation decreases with continued use, as the hairs growing back are distributed more sparsely and are finer in texture. Epilady can be purchased at most major department stores. For further information, call 1-800-444-LEGS.

More Camouflage

If there are personal traits with which you are dissatisfied, there are ways to camouflage them. For example, if your hip is high, or perhaps uneven, arm movements can obscure that fact. You can adjust your stance to camouflage such traits as bowed legs, knock-knees and foot problems. If you have very thin calves or too much space showing between your legs, turning your front ankle in slightly can be attractive and help camouflage these figure faults. "Knobby knees" look best either bent or with one ankle arched next to the other. Girls with either "knobby knees" or skinny legs should never stand completely in profile. In the swimsuit stance, holding one arm slightly further back near the hip can help disguise "fanny overhand." Donna Lee advises, "Earrings may be used to attract attention to the face thereby distracting from heavy hips or bottoms. However, I am cautious when I see a girl trying deliberately to distract me — I begin to look for the problem area." To embellish small lips or draw attention to the mouth, choose a light glossy shade of lipstick. To de-emphasize the mouth, wear a dark lipstick with a matte finish. If you have a round face, you can give the illusion that is slimmer by tilting your head to the left or right, displaying your most flattering side. The tilted angle accentuates cheekbones, flattens protruding ears and exposes your hairstyle dimensions. If you tilt your head forward, your chin and jaw line will appear smaller.

Rarely are a girl's proportions the same on the left and right sides. Because of this, you want to avoid hitting the judges head-on. Avoiding the situation, however, may be impossible. If you are in this type of agonizing dilemma, heed Mary Francis Flood's advice, "... in the manner of your walk, the way you throw your arms, and the sparkle in your eyes as well as the beautiful smile on your face, you can hide your flaws." No one is perfect, so minimize your imperfections and remember, they are never as obvious to others as they are to you.

Critiquing Yourself

In order to polish these aspects of a more pleasing appearance that will enhance your looks, it is wise to look critically at yourself as a whole — hair, skin, body, hands, apparel, grooming, makeup and personality. You need to work from head to toe on every detail, concentrating on smoothing away any rough ages. Only then can you begin to reach your goals. The wise contestant is one who adds up her physical, emotional, and spiritual assets on a continuing basis and pays attention to those elements that need work. If you intend to be a beauty queen, any response less then "great" won't do!

To make changes, you need definite guidelines. If you don't know how to exercise or eat properly, many books are written on these subjects. If you are having difficulties in controlling compulsive eating habits, there is help available. I'm often asked asked how professional models stay trim. Most models to who I spoke to said they didn't diet, but they did make it a point to eat sensibly. Many restricted their fat intake. Some admitted to "falling off the wagon once in a while and eating a banana split every so often," but they also quickly resumed their healthy schedule. The Food Addiction Hot Line, sponsored by the Florida Institute of Technology, provides free support for compulsive overeaters as well as information on where to get help in your area. For further information, call their toll-free number 1-800-USA-0088.

You need to take responsibility to keep fit. When you make progress, even if it is not to your "ideal" weight, have a positive attitude. You don't have to have a perfect body to be able to say, "I like how I look and feel." *Ideal*, like *success*, is not easy to define.

Buying Yourself

The goal of this preparation is to be ready to "sell" yourself to the judges. Before you can sell yourself to anyone else, you must sell yourself *to yourself*. For many girls, this is the hardest part. Remember, people will accept you at your own valuation. If you don't think well of yourself, no one else will either. Unless you believe in your own ability, you can't convince others of it.

A self-improvement program should be based on balance. As with anything else, it is not good to overdo exercising and dieting. We've all encountered people who talk incessantly about their figure problems, hairstyles, or their fight against cellulite to the exclusion of every other topic of conversation. Being obsessed with looks can destroy the possibility of being well rounded — or well liked.

At the same time, sometimes you have to work at liking yourself. If you've decided to make the very best of yourself and to develop all those positive aspects of your good looks, then you are a winner for having focused on the 80% positive rather than the 20% that's negative. Spotlight your good points. Feeling good about yourself gives you the energy and the will-power to improve upon the negatives. If you do not have the body of an athlete or the face of a princess, keep reminding yourself of what you do have. If people compliment you on your wonderful personality, you have the greatest compensatory factor of all. In fact, many "beautiful" people would gladly change places with you, so rather than feel sorry for yourself, look for ways to highlight your asset. It's easy to see that you don't have to be born with perfect features and a perfect body to make yourself look attractive. There are enough choices at the cosmetic counter to help any girl make the most of her natural assets. Just learn to accentuate the positive and *listen* when people tell you how beautiful you are. Believe in yourself and never second-guess your decisions. There are no limits to what you can do. Just keep working toward your goal, and *don't give up* when it's something you want.

The Self-Awareness Notebook

You can begin your self-improvement program with a self-awareness notebook. Keep your self-awareness notebook to monitor your personal goals. Write down what needs to be done to improve your appearance or self-confidence, for example. You are not stuck with your present degree of confidence. Confidence can be developed if you work hard at it. Keeping this notebook will allow you to keep track of the things you do for yourself. You can refer to it periodically and see where you need more attention. Your self-awareness notebook should also state resolutions, a timetable for meeting goals, a clear description of the means by which you plan to achieve them, and an evaluation of your progress. If you want to lose weight, for example, paste an old snapshot of yourself when you were an ideal weight at the beginning of the notebook.

Below are suggestions for enclosures in your notebook and for a format to use:

Steps to believing in yourself:

1. Emphasize the positive: "Sure my eyelid twitched, but I looked

nice in the interview."

2. Recognize that you are not the only center of attention. The chances are small that the audience were WATCHING your feet to notice that your shoe came off when you were walking.

3. Learn not to jump to conclusions. Jumping to conclusions is a two part error. It combines mind reading with fortune telling. Practice focusing your attention so completely, that your mind does not have time to draw conclusions. If you practice complicated breathing routines or thought patterns, you can remain much more confident while you finish your competition.

4. Set reasonable expectations for yourself. You won't become Miss Somebody overnight. However, your chances improve when you put your heart into the matter and work on your faults. If you need to become more comfortable speaking to a group of people, ITC (formerly International Toastmistress) is an organization that helps people improve their communication skills. It also teaches you how to organize your thoughts logically and to present them with self-assurance. This increases your confidence. You can write to ITC Headquarters, 9068 East Firestone Boulevard, Suite 2, Downey, CA 90241, to find the name and meeting place of a group near you.

5. Know your good points. Instead of focusing on negatives, focus on the positive things about yourself. If you have big feet, focus attention on your legs.

6. Please yourself. Do not enter a pageant in order to please others. If you do not win a pageant that you entered for another person, you will have failed. If you do not win a pageant that you entered for yourself, you will have won because of the positive experiences you had by participating.

7. Seek small victories. Pat yourself on the back for having entered the pageant, rather than berating yourself for not being the titleholder. Having entered is a victory. Recognize the extra poise and confidence you have gained for the rest of your life.

8. Reward yourself. Whether or not you are the titleholder, enjoy your success. When you have completed pageant, take yourself — and others — out to a movie. When you get positive feedback, treat yourself to a luncheon or an outfit you've been wanting.

9. Regard mistakes as stepping stones on the path to wisdom.

Learn from your mistakes; don't dwell on them or let them drag you down. Be glad you have learned those lessons and don't have to repeat them. Nevertheless, give yourself permission to make some mistakes. Allowing yourself to be less than perfect gives you the freedom to be at ease.

10. Practice using positive terms in daily conversations, sounding confident. For example, no matter what internal doubts you may have, speak without hedges. Avoid "but," "maybe," or "I'm not sure." These words imply negative feelings. When you are firmly convinced that you are going to become the next Miss Somebody, you are halfway there.

11. Look confident. Everyday, dress and groom yourself to show that you are feeling on top of the world — whether you are or not. Stand as if you are an inch taller and walk with a firm, purposeful stride. When you keep your head up and walk confidently, you build your self-confidence.

12. Initiate conversations, especially with people you do not know. The more you do this, the easier it becomes. People with whom you strike up a conversation are unlikely to turn and run away or act insulted that you noticed them. Similarly, starting the conversation with another contestant at a pageant function will build your confidence. Additionally, that person will generally respond with interest and gratitude, and you will have won a friend.

13. Imitate self-confident people. When you look and act self-confident, people will treat you as if you are. There is nothing to stroke the ego like being treated like someone to emulate. It becomes a self-fulfilling prophecy. When you note and imitate the attractions of confident people, you increase your own capabilities.

14. Take a self-survey. Write comments on the condition of your:

Hair
Styling _____
Color _____
Scalp and hair condition _____

Face
Skin _____
Appropriateness of your makeup palette _____
Makeup application skills _____
Shape of your eyebrows _____

Body

osture _____
ody shape and weight distribution _____
Skin texture, tone, blemishes, trouble spots _____
Hands and fingernails _____
Feet and toenails _____

15. Weight chart. Keep a chart in which you record your weight periodically. Buy some gold start and paste them on your chart as you reach intermediate goals.

16. Measurement chart. Make a record weekly of your measurements, awarding yourself gold stars as you reduce or enlarge those measurements that do not meet your expectations.

"Stage Fright"

"Stage fright" prevents many people from speaking or appearing in front of a large group. It is often worse if your performance is being critiqued or graded for competition. "Combating stage fright and nerves comes with continuing to compete," says Kelli Lee. You can learn to combat anxiety by promoting relaxation. By learning deep muscle relaxation, you will be able to relax beyond your usual ability.

Deep Muscle Relaxation

Practice deep muscle relaxation at least twice a day for a minimum of two weeks prior to your pageant. Become aware of which muscle groups are harder for you to relax. For instance, some people find that their abdominal and back muscles are constantly tensed. Learn to relax all your muscle groups, especially those that are usually tensed. Once your body does not have to cope with tensed muscles, it will have more energy to concentrate on the situation at hand. This is healthier and will usually lead to a more successful outcome. You alleviate anxiety more effectively by doing something — i.e. relaxation. Books which can teach you to combat stress and anxiety include Michele Haney and Edmond W. Boenish's *StressMap: Finding Your Pressure Points* and *The Relaxation and Stress Reduction Workbook* by Martha Davis, Matthew McKay and Elizabeth Robbins.

Proper Breathing Techniques

Proper breathing techniques also help promote relaxation. When you inhale, the muscle that separates your lungs from your abdomen, that is your diaphragm, should stretch, allowing the lungs to expand downward. When you exhale, the diaphragm should again push up against the lungs, expelling the air.

Unfortunately, when we are tense, we breathe shallowly. That keeps the diaphragm from doing its job effectively. When you are not getting enough oxygen, because you are breathing inefficeintly, and you are anxious, you breathe more rapidly — to get more oxygen. This leads to an upset in the balance of oxygen and carbon dioxide in the blood. This imbalance is called hyperventilation, and it creates muscle tension, especially in the neck and shoulders. It can also cause chest pains and headaches.

It is possible to learn a more relaxed breathing rate. First, establish your current rate. Count the number of breaths you take in one minute. If this number is greater than 13, you have room for improvement in your breathing technique. Next look at your chest and abdomen. If your chest moves when you breathe, but your abdomen doesn't, this is another sign that you are not breathing right.

Breathe through your nose rather than through your mouth, both to slow down your rate and to decrease the volume of air that you swallow rather than utilize. To exhale properly, pull in your stomach slightly at the end of each exhalation. In hale by just letting your lungs slowly fill with air. It should take at least eight seconds to fully inflate your lungs. Do not consciously inhale.

Karyl Gammon, publisher of the *Arizona Pageant Update*, suggests the following to combat nerves before appearing on stage: "Next time you are waiting in the wings to go on stage, with your arms at your side, make a fist and squeeze as hard as you can. Then take three deep breaths and release just before going on stage. This helps to release a lot of nervous tension and allows you to relax and look more natural."

Your Aural Face

Your voice is your aural face. It is almost as important to your ɔearance as your eyes and your smile. "The tone of your voice aunost is more important than your skin, your hair, and your eyes," says Jane Jaffe. "Voice inflection is probably on of the most important things I teach at John Robert Powers. For example, a very high-pitched voice will be very unpleasant to listen to. And not only is it unpleasant, it gives one the impression that this is an uneducated person. A whiny voice says that this is not a mature person, that she wants to stay a little girl." High-pitched voices indicate nervousness and insecurity, not to mention being very irritating to listeners. Low tones convey competence. Donna Lee says, "I can tell a lot about a contestant by her tone of voice. I can detect nervousness, insincerity, insecurity and merely being unable to handle making appearances. To me, a mousy voice indicates a mousy personality." Evaluate and polish your voice by speaking into a tape recorder. Analyze your voice, gauging its volume, noting the rate and pace of your speech. It should be at a moderate level and neither too fast nor too slow. For your most effective voice, keep your shoulders back and your spine straight. Slouching causes your voice to sound reedy and apathetic. Jane Jaffe recommends diction lessons for serious pageant contestants.

Posture

Your posture onstage is crucial. Never show any trace of swayback. Hold your head high with your chin parallel to the ground. Your shoulders should be back and down, your chest up, and your elbows slightly bent. Your upper body should be straight, the shoulders and torso angled slightly to the side for a slimmer, taller line. Be sure that one shoulder is not higher than the other — in the classic shoulder bag hunch. Your hands should be relaxed and still, and your finger tips should lightly touch your legs. Lisa Jaffe, *Miss Mid City* 1987 recommends, "If your hands are not relaxed naturally, touch the tip of your thumb to the middle joint of your middle finger and hold it there."

Judging Criteria

In the swimsuit and evening gown competitions you will stand in full front standing position. You will be judged according to conformance to the following points:

1) An imaginary line through the center of your head must pass

through your torso, dividing your legs, with pressure evenly distributed on both legs.

2) Your neck must be graceful enough to act as a pedestal for your head. This can be accomplished by using the back muscles of your neck, keeping your head up.

3) Your shoulders must be wider than your hips and slope at a 20 degree angle from the base of your neck.

4) Your arms must flow as you stand or walk.

5) Your legs must be elegant when standing and graceful when walking. Calf muscles should be evenly distributed. Half of the weight should be on the inside toe border, the other half should be on the outside.

The Miss America Walk

The *Miss America* walk is the Suck-and-Tuck Glide. You suck in your stomach and tuck in your derriere, walking briskly. At the same time, you swing your arms in time with the alternate legs. This helps to mask big thighs. In the swimsuit, stand so that no light shines between your legs. The only two spaces permitted are below the knees and at the ankles. Stand in the basic pageant stance so that your legs are together. When properly executed, this elongates and slims your body and legs. Once you are onstage, pause at the center until it seems you have everyone looking at you. Do not proceed forward until you feel you have everyone's attention. Prior to stepping forward, take several deep breaths so you can build every to move to the next point on stage. Look natural, don't hurry to your next position, maintain eye contact with the judges, and enjoy your moment.

The Pivot

A pivot is the method of changing your point of direction. Pageant contestants use the same pivot that models use. A pivot, either full or half, is executed from the pageant stance. Begin with the front foot leading and your weight centered on the back. This leaves the front foot free to move forward. Take two small steps, with the feet pointing straight ahead, starting with the front food. Stop, shifting your weight to the balls of your feet. Turn in a half circle so that you are now facing in the opposite direction. Shift your weight to the back foot; this completes a half pivot. To complete a full pivot, your head does not turn with the body. Instead, it follows, giving a slight over-the-shoulder look. On the second half of the turn, your head can turn with the body. When pivoting, turn slowly. As Christy Cole notes, "Whirling around quickly doesn't give the judges a good look at what you really have under your hood!"

Sometimes, your walk and pivot are choreographed and marks are placed on the stage for you to "hit." Donna Lee does not like this system because contestants my "seem tentative because they may miss a mark." Barbara Kelley recommends that if you have to stop at specific locations you should "'spot' your 'mark' about 4 feet from it, so you stop gracefully." To do so, glance down with only your eyes, keeping your head up and your chin parallel to the ground. Never tilt your head. Similarly, if you must negotiate stairs, execute the maneuver with your body turned slightly sideways. If there is a rail, glide one hand lightly on it. The angled torso prevents the "all knees" look. When you descend a stairway, keep your knees slightly bent to avoid bouncing. You can also use the professional modeling trick — count the number of steps you will step down in advance. No matter what "tips" you use, practice until your moves are smooth and graceful.

Correcting Your Posture

Posture is the single most important word in your body language. Rounded shoulders project shyness and diffidence, while perfect posture mirrors a positive attitude and healthy self-esteem. When you walk proudly, but not stiffly, erect, you are telling the world that you are an important person in your own right. Clothes look best on people who have good posture and walk with grace. When you hold yourself well, inexpensive clothes become expensive-looking. If you feel your posture needs improvement, a posture therapist can help you.

One such posture therapist is Bernice Danylchuk of La Jolla, California. Bernice developed Physio-Dynamics, a method of therapeutic posture realignment. She advises, "A person does not have to endure the discomfort or mental anguish of bow legs, round shoulders, dowager's hump, caved-in chest with attendant breathing problems or low back pain." Bernice teaches, "The human body does not achieve alignment and good posture naturally. It must be informed by the mind. Properly trained, the mind directs the nerves which transmit messages to muscles and ligaments. Then these powerful muscles and ligaments align the bone structure for healthful posture in standing, walking, sitting, squatting, lifting, bending and running. Together with proper breathing, the body can then be restored to youthful agility."

A Danylchuk posture session is different from any other. you start out before a mirror with Bernice barking instructions at you as though she were a drill sergeant. Skillfully, she takes you through stances, stretches and exercises to show you what it feels like when your "wings" are together in back and your pelvis, chin, knees and back are all tilted at just the right angles. With her assistant, Toby Danylchuk, Bernice helps relax muscles and break down holding patterns by "walking" on you with bare feet. She kneads your arms, legs, chest and thighs while you lie on a floor mat. It's all strange and different, but it works.

Perhaps Bernices' most dramatic achievement came with a teen-age boy named Kyle Sager who flew to La Jolla from Georgia to see if Bernice could correct a severe posture problem. "He was bow-legged and walked on the sides of his fee," recalls Bernice. "The doctors said nothing could be done." After 13 lessons, with Bernice coaxing Kyle to use his leg muscles properly and straightening out his poor body alignment, his awkward gait was corrected. "When his parents saw him walk off the plane, they couldn't believe he was their son."

Bernice remembers the rehearsals of *Lipstick*. According to her recollection, film actress Margaux Hemingway was unable to walk gracefully in one costume — a heavy beaded dress. It only took four lessons to take the "clumsiness" out of Margaux Hemingway's movements. Other celebrity clients who have benefited from Physio-Dynamics include Burt Reynolds, Burgess Meredith, Cloris Leachman, Carroll O'Connor, and Olympic diver Greg Louganis.

Bernice Danylchuk's Physio-Dynamics has helped MD's, yogis, academicians, and pageant officials, as well as pageant contestants. Bernice, herself, is considered a genius at body alignment.

San Diego pageant contestant Elizabeth Leavell says Bernice is "God-sent." For further information about Physio-Dynamics, see Appendix G.

A Pageant Where Everyone Wins

Edison Technical High School in Fresno, California conducts a pageant each year. The physical education teacher rates each contestant according to the following point scale:

	Points
I. Posture 60	
1. Walking	20
2. Sitting	20
3. Plumb line	20
II. Teeth 60	
1. Condition	30
2. Cleanliness	30
III. Nails 60	
1. Condition of cuticle	
2. Cleanliness	
IV. Hair 60	
1. Cleanliness of hair	20
2. Cleanliness of scalp	20
3. General appearance	20
V. Skin 60	
1. Cleanliness	30
2. Lack of imperfection	30
VI. Muscle Tone 20	
1. Firmness of muscles	
VII. Motor Ability 60	
1. Walk	6
2. Run	6
3. Skip	6
4. Hop	6
5. Jump	6
6. Balance	6
7. Bend	6

8. Catch	6	
9. Throw	6	
10. Sit	6	

VIII. General Appearance 60

1. Neatness of dress	20
2. Symmetry of form	20
3. General cleanliness	20

IX. Weight

Weight Scale

Percentage overweight	Points	Percentage underweight
2 to 4	55	2 to 3
5 to 6	50	4 to 5
7 to 8	40	5
9 to 10	30	6
10	20	7
15	10	10
20	5	20

The six or seven girls who score highest are presented to the student assembly as the titleholders of the contest. Honorable mention awards are given to those having scored above 400 points. Obviously, everyone entering this contest leaves it as a winner.

Chapter 4

POLISHING YOUR COMPETITIVE PERSONA

Public relations is not only a big part of a titleholder's responsibilities, but the communication skills used in those public relations are important in gaining the title. Consequently, contestants should hone their communication skills. Communication is an exchange, so cultivate an awareness of how the other party is receiving your message, how they are likely to react.

Listen Carefully

Listen carefully, rather than composing your next statement. You can only learn by listening to what is actually being said. Mary Francis Flood notes, "In order to communicate well, you must listen intently. Then you're not likely to be misunderstood. Never speak hastily. You need to listen intently before you answer someone's question." Be interested instead of trying to be interesting. Having listened carefully, you will know what to say, because you will know what was asked.

Establish and Maintain Eye Contact

Another prerequisite to good communication skills is establishing and maintaining eye contact. Do not look down or away from the person speaking, and never focus on a spot somewhere over the speaker's shoulder. Hold a direct, clear gaze, allowing your eyes to express that you are interested in what the speaker is saying.

Know Your Language

Misusing the language is a bad mistake. Do not use words whose meaning you don't know. It is difficult to be in control of your meaning, if you're not in control of the words. Use the language correctly, avoiding slang, superlatives and "popular" phrases. Be direct, smooth and articulate. When you are asked what characteristics you *possess*, the correct response is a noun naming that trait. If you are asked for a word that *describes* you, respond with an adjective. Being precise in your use of language will impress the judges.

Current Events

Be prepared to discuss current events, for the interview competition, for pop questions and for media interviews following your crowning. After you are crowned it will be too late to prepare. Reading the newspaper and news magazines like *Time*, *Newsweek*, or *U.S. News and World Report*, will help you know current events, while watching *60 Minutes*, *20/20*, and the morning interview shows like *CBS This Morning*, *Good Morning America*, and *Today* will show what is topical. One former *Miss Arizona* took a more direct approach. She wrote directly to ABC's *Nightline* to ask for information about the Iran-Contra Hearings. They sent her, in response, the exact questions that had been asked — *and* the answers. If you need direction in staying informed, you may wish to find a current events coach. They can guide you and translate world events into a form more easily understood.

A Caring, Friendly Demeanor

Yet another aspect of communication skills is projecting a caring, friendly demeanor. Demonstrate yours by extending the smile of friendship to those with whom you are competing. The pageant path is a long, winding one. Contestants work hard and deserve to be encouraged by their fellow competitors as well as by sponsors, friends and families. You are in a unique position to understand and support each other, and the pageant will be more fun for all if you devote your energies to building camaraderie rather than envy or jealousy. At coronation time, gather around the newly chosen queen and extend your appreciation to her. She worked as hard as you did and deserves your positive support. Besides, this is a chance to perfect your poise under stress — the very traits that may carry the day for you, the next time out.

Perhaps the hardest part of graciousness and public relations is accepting with appreciation the hard work and support that others give to us. It is often much easier to work hard and support another than it is to smile gratefully and say thank you. At the same time, it is essential to not lose sight of the fact that others are giving us the *gifts* of support and hard work. We do not deserve them by *right*. Nothing attains perfection, neither people or pageants, but many people work very hard and give a great deal so that contestants have the opportunity to enrich their lives through a pageant program.

Laugh At Yourself

Learn to laugh at yourself and with others. Develop and keep a good sense of humor, whatever the situation. No situation is so bad that there is not a laugh buried somewhere in it. The trick is to look for it and appreciate it. Contestants should expect to make mistakes, and they should learn to be at ease with failure. Expect to be involved in embarrassing situations. This will help you survive the situation, even if you cannot immediately see the humor. A friend tells me that her husband told her that they had been invited to a military Christmas party. This friend went out to buy the perfect party dress. When she didn't find the "right" dress, she decided to take advantage of the informality of parties in Hawaii and wear a muumuu in Christmas colors. Imagine her feelings when she walked into the "party," to discover that this was a military ball and every other woman was wearing an evening gown! She says it was only her sense of the ridiculous, plus the certainty that *someday* it would be a funny story, that got her through the interminable evening. Pageants are a hurry up and wait game. Expect to be bored, scared, on top of the world, and so low that the bottom looks up. Through it all, you must keep your sense of humor and smile — no matter what!

Good Manners

Good manners are based on a genuine concern for others. Good manners reflect upon you, your family, your friends and your background. People judge not only the individual but also that individual's family by the way she acts. The importance of good manners can never be overestimated. They shine in your approach to life. Instill in yourself the values of honesty, helpfulness and caring. If you get into habits of deceiving yourself and being blind to the needs of others, you will become alienated from yourself. Remain true to the best that is in you, and the rest will fall into place. This is the key to success. Contestants who are honestly helpful and giving towards others are the ones who fare best in competition. In the 1985 *Miss Coastal Bend* pageant, one contestant asked another to help her pin up her hair for competition. A third contestant recognized the poor job that the second had done and redid the styling for the first contestant. Everyone was pleased when this thoughtful contestant was crowned the winner.

The Right Attitude

Approach each pageant with the right attitude and maintain it whether you win or lose. "Optimism and humor are a contestant's most important quality," says Barbara Kelley. "I also look for a girl who's unique." Adopt the attitude that you are a winner and that you are bound to win maturity, a better understanding of people, a pride in your accomplishments and a consciousness of your own beauty, both inward and outward.

Competition should always be free of petty ego, vanity, selfishness, greed and bad manners. It should be friendly, helpful and giving. Once you lose a grip on reality, you also lose a grip on your own self-worth. The purpose of competition is to provide an opportunity for self-objectivity, as well as a means to channel talents. Unselfish contestants realize that it is an honor and a responsibility to be a contestant, that good sportsmanship is vital to competition and that winning is unimportant. The pageant itself is the stepping-stone in developing their character and future. Barbara Kelley says, "Life is competitive. The more practice we have, the better our chances are of being successful."

Be nice to everyone you meet, not just to people you think can help you. Imagine how mortified you would be to meet the gentleman you snubbed in the lobby sitting on the judges panel in the interview room! The members of the pageant committee, for example, may never cross your path again, while you'll be surprised to find someone helps you out later — even much later — just because he or she was the recipient of your kindness. I met a gentleman at a library one day and discovered he was the host of a San Diego TV show only when he invited me to appear on a segment of that show. You only have one chance to make a first impression, and for better or worse, that impression will remain permanently on file in that person's memory bank. It's nice to be important, but it's more important to be nice. This positive attitude of honesty, helping and caring — niceness — is your greatest asset. It conveys confidence and radiates happiness.

Priorities

Contestants have been known to lose track of their priorities or, worse, set inappropriate ones once they enter a pageant. Keep your priorities in order at all times, especially when competing in pageants. Do not forget those who have helped you get to where you currently are. Remember to send thank you notes within two weeks of the end of the pageant to your sponsors as well as to anyone who sent you gifts or flowers. "Write a special note to your parents and friends who helped, encouraged, paid for, and cried through this wonderful time with you," says Jane Jaffe. You would not be in the pageant without the support of your family and sponsors. "It takes so little to be above average," reminds Lisa Jaffe, *Miss Mid City* 1987.

A titleholder is a symbol of beauty and grace, and she must keep this in mind during the year she reigns. Once chosen, she must not relax just because the pressure of competition is off. She is in the spotlight — the symbol of what her pageant system represents. There is no excuse for a titleholder to let any aspect of her winning persona to get out of shape.

In order to perform well in a pageant, you have to have a single vision. By that, I mean you can't have three goals going at once. You can't simultaneously compete in a pageant, spend time with your friends, and be with your boyfriend. If you are doing three things at once, you won't be able to do any of them well. Jane Jaffe notes, "If you decide you want to win a pageant, then that has to be your focus and your goal, and you have to be single-minded about it. There are a lot of people who are going to be negative when you say you're entering pageants. There will be family and friends and boyfriends who don't want you to do this. They don't want you to do it for a lot of reasons. Some of them will be jealous; some of them are frightened. They think if you win this pageant you'll be a different person. Boyfriends especially are not good about wanting their girlfriends to be in pageants because they want their undivided attention." Being in a pageant is time-consuming. You will have to exercise, practice walking, and practice interview technique. You're going to spend your free time preparing for the pageant. That means you won't have time to be going out with boyfriends or girlfriends. "If your priority isn't to win the pageant, you see, you will not win the pageant because you'll spend the time with your friends instead," warns Jane. "You have to decide how much you really want this. If you're just starting out in pageants or whether you're going to a state or national pageant, there is a certain amount of time you're going to have to devote."

Winning and Losing

Despite the time you spend in preparation, only one contestant will win the title. If that contestant is not you, you will still be a winner for having competed. You will have learned to present yourself in a positive manner. Mary Francis Flood advises, "Not to win is not a sin, but not to try is a tragedy. If you have faith in yourself, there is nothing in this world that can keep you from achieving any goal that you set yourself. Many people try to have a life of no hits, no runs, no errors. They never try to do anything, but if you try, you will succeed."

When it's time to announce the semifinalists, do not lose your professional attitude. If you did not make the cut, a good outlook will help you through the feelings of rejection. Do not feel that you let your entire hometown down. You should reason, "I gave it a good shot. Next time ..." DO NOT CRY. It is distressing to see someone feeling so sorry for herself. "Losing a pageant causes a lot of soul searching," says Kelli Lee. "I always try to examine what I did while competing. If I find no answer, I do realize that judging is a matter of personal opinion and obviously I wasn't their choice." Furthermore, "There is absolutely nothing more reward-ing than when I know that I have done my best job and I deserve the title. I do feel, however, that you can win too much and that sometimes you must lose in order to win."

"I don't have to have a crown to be a winner," Brandi Gammon told her mother after losing a pageant. Brandi's mom, Karyl Gammon, editor and publisher of the *Arizona Pageant Update*, says, "With each pageant experience you will make new friends and gain more confidence and poise. Go into the competition with the idea that you will do the best you can do and to have a good time. When you no longer enjoy competing, you should quit." You don't have to win a pageant to be a winner for life.

A Second Try

A common question is "Should I give a pageant a second try?" The decision is even more difficult if you have previously placed as a runner up. Returning as last year's runner-up places you in an awkward position. The other contestants are bound to see you as a strong participant. You must realize that, no matter what the contestants' perceptions, doing well in the past does not ensure doing well on your next try. This judging panel is different from last year's panel, and they may be seeking something very dif-ferent in the winner they choose than last year's panel was seek-ing.

Title winners have to consider whether or not they should com-pete again for a title they have already held. Kelli Lee says, "I do not feel that a girl who presently holds the title being sought by others should be allowed to compete for the title again. I have no problem, however, with the girl returning after a year's layoff. I personally would not compete for a title because I use pageants as goals. Once I achieve a goal, I feel that it is time to move on to other goals."

Who Wins Beauty Pageants?

In general, the questions you have about who wins beauty pageants are reflections of your areas of insecurity and indications of aspects you should work on prior to entering a pageant. How-ever, there is an overall characterization to these questions, and the answers reinforce the fact that judges are not look for a kind of girl, they are seeking a girl who is the best she can be.

Could a girl win a pageant without winning any preliminary events? Kylene Barker, *Miss Virginia*, was considered a long-shot for the title because she had not won any of the preliminary competitions. Even so, she did become *Miss America* 1979. It is better to be strong in *all* aspects of competition, rather than a preliminary winner in one area and ho-hum in another.

Does a girl need to be well endowed to win a beauty pageant? Bustlines do not win pageants, girls do. It takes more than a large bustline to win pageants. Concentrate on improving your natural assets instead of worrying about what you might lack. Your bustline does not determine who you are or what you can achieve.

Do blondes/brunettes/redheads win more pageants? There is no single standard of beauty in pageants. In the 1988 *Miss Universe* pageant, all the finalists were brunettes. On the other hand, *Miss USA* 1988 was a blonde.

Do you have to be tall to win a beauty pageant? When asked if a woman 5'3" could win the title, George Honchar, president of *Miss Universe*, Inc., responded, "Sure, because if she did, she'd be an incredible 5'3"."[1] The truth of this was demonstrated when Barbara Palacios Teyde, 5'2", was crowned *Miss Universe* 1986. Gretchen Carlson, *Miss America* 1989, stands 5'3". She is the shortest titleholder in that system since Margaret Gorman, *Miss America* 1921. Miss Gorman was 5'1". Kylene Barker, *Miss America* 1979, and Susan Powell, *Miss America* 1981, were both 5'4". Viewers discern height by comparison. It is, therefore, much more important for body parts to be in proportion to each other than that you be any particular height.

What if all the other contestants are more beautiful than I am? It takes more than beautiful looks to win a beauty pageant. In fact, you must not depend on your looks to win. Beauty begins from within. Pageants are not seeking just drop-dead-gorgeous contestants. Leonard Horn, the *Miss America* pageant director, advises, "If a young woman considered herself to be the ugliest person in the

1   *People*, July 15, 1985

world, she could still enter a local pageant. Those who enter these contests enter because they are confident enough of their beauty. So what is defined as 'beauty' is self-limiting by the contestants."[2] According to a 1987 study in *The Harper's Index*, only about 13 percent of American women consider themselves to be pretty. This misperception is what Mr. Horn means by beauty being self-limiting.

Will my chances be better if I change my name? If you would feel better by changing your name, then do so. However, a girl's changing her name does not improve her chances at winning the crown. In 1945, Lenora Slaughter, executive director of the *Miss America* pageant, suggested that one contestant change her name. She thought that Betty Merrick would be a better show business name. The contestant did not take her advice, and despite that Bess Myerson went on to be *Miss America* 1945.

Should I have surgery to perfect my body for the pageant? Surgery is always risky; it is a decision that should be made with your doctor, for your life, not for a beauty pageant. Having surgery to make a feature conform to an aesthetic ideal does not enhance your chances to win the pageant. Beauty comes from within, not from without. It takes time to recover from surgery, perhaps as much time as it would take to work on the "flaw" without surgery. "If a girl needs lots of work on her body to get it in tip-top shape, I would say it takes for most girls approximately three months," says Mary Francis Flood. "And again, this is going to determine what areas of the body a girl is working on. Does she need thigh reduction? Does she need bust development? Does she need to tone the arms? Does she need to build the calves up? Perhaps down? The length of time depends upon the contestant."

Do Southern girls have an advantage in national competitions? Have you ever noticed how a girl becomes more beautiful the minute her name is announced as queen and the crown is placed on her head? Feeling like a beauty queen causes her to have a more self-confident appearance. In the South, being a beauty queen is something that a girl's aunt or mother has done, it is an image with which young women grow up. Adding to that, pageants are an industry in the South. Because there are more pageants available to them and they have had more exposure to pageantry, the odds are increased that a Southern contestant will be relaxed and comfortable when she reaches the national level. However, despite the run of five consecutive *Miss USAs* from Texas, the long term statistics for both *Miss America* and *Miss USA* do not support the contention that Southern belles have a competitive edge.

Hallmarks of a Winner

A beauty queen is America's number one symbol of sweetness, femininity and wholesome good looks as well as a role model for the young women in this country. She is a symbol of innocence, what America represents. Keep this image alive by presenting yourself in the best possible manner. Clean living and hard effort can spell success for you; and should you win, your crown will not be tarnished.

The hallmarks of a true beauty pageant winner are:
- playing within the bounds of fair competition
- reacting with grace after making a mistake
- believing in herself
- being frank without being offensive
- holding family relationships ahead of winning
- refusing to step on other people in order to win
- maintaining her gracious attitude when another wins the title
- meaning it when she says, "May the best girl win"
- thoroughly preparing for all aspects of competition
- undertaking her responsibilities with pride
- helping and encouraging others.

A true winner is made, she is not born; she has a dream, and she works to make it happen. The dream of every contestant in a pageant is to be the ONE girl who is crowned the winner. By definition, she is unique. Part of your goal, then, is demonstrating your uniqueness, not only in your appearance, but also in your demeanor. Make friends with contestants, but don't become part of a clique — be an individual. The best way to stand out, of course, is simply not to worry about winning and simply enjoy the pageant for its own sake. This attitude will relax you, so you won't have to *try* to impress the judges. Believing that you will perform at a higher level than your competitors frees you from having to be anxious, second-guess yourself in relation to other contestants, and worry about technical aspect of competition. Believing you are capable of winning, and in fact, believing you are the best contestant out there gives you the competitive edge. A self-assured person is intimidating to others, particularly those who are not self-assured. If you let yourself become intimidated, on the other hand, you risk losing your self-assurance, and your performance will suffer — to the benefit of your self-assured opponents. Enjoy competing and cultivate the "gut" feeling that you are going to win. It is as possible to have positive "gut" feelings as to have negative ones.

A Competitive Edge

As mentioned previously, every contestant wants to be the one crowned the queen. So, every contestant is seeking a "competitive edge." That competitive edge is simple: Know the system. You don't have to be sophisticated, glamorous, or wealthy to be a beauty queen. Knowing the system, you'll be that much closer to the crown of your dreams. A good way to learn about the system is simply by entering pageants.

Part of the agricultural heritage of this country is the tradition of harvest festivals. Each of these, as well as the Country and State fairs provide an opportunity to become experienced in pageantry. Far from being disadvantageous to be the graduate of such "small town" competitions, being from a close-knit community provides a support system that is hard to beat. The strivings of a local contestant are as important to a girl's neighbor as they are to her family. When a girls from a small town enters a state or national pageant, the entire town supports her 110% of the way.

The best advice I can give you is to be prepared for competition. Do not be afraid to ask for assistance from your friends, parents, modeling instructors, dance teachers, or your pageant director. View pageants as positive growing experiences. Karen Kemple advises, "Try entering as many pageant competitions, at various levels, and as often as possible. They can act as proving grounds for future competitions." She also recommends learning from valuable insights of friends who have had pageant experience.

Enter pageants as a self-improvement course and be willing to work and apply yourself. "Think like a winner, give it your best shot, learn from your mistakes and work to improve one hundred percent," says Barbara Kelley. "Enter again and again. The Champion's Creed says, 'I'm not judged by the number of times I succeed, but by the number of times I fail and keep trying to do better!' Above all, have fun! Go in a contest and learn; if you win, that's icing on the cake." Winning a pageant does take work, so prepare yourself well for pageant competition. Mary Francis Flood comments, "If you prepare yourself well, enter pageant, and don't win, then you say 'Lord, I did the best I could. I ran a good race. Thank you, Lord, for being with me. I know you have something for me along the road you want me to do.'"

Making A Good Competition Better

You *can* help to make a good competition better by taking a few minutes to thin. Be on your toes, look alert and know when it's your turn to compete. Help other competitors get ready for the competition. Enjoy what is going on around you. Meet new friends and seek out new ideas and methods. Remember that you are important to pageantry. Without contestants — even the one who finishes last — there is no pageant. The winner's star shines briefly. Savor the moment and get on with life.

Don't be embarrassed if you do not win. The successful contestant accepts her mistakes, appraising them realistically. She feels that she belongs and deserves to be in the competition. The world will accept you at your own evaluation. If you expect the world to watch for a chance to jeer at you, they will, and you will be embarrassed. Those who are self-assured are resistant to such concerns; they continue to recognize that they belong — even if they did not perform well this time out.

A girl must prepare to lose with dignity, as well as to win with humility. "If you don't win, then someone else more deserving did win and maybe the timing was not right for you. Look at the judges and say 'Thank you' whether or not you win because it is very important to have a good attitude. For some girls, in order to seek a crown, they have to go back several times in the same pageant in order to accomplish their goal. Or perhaps they are supposed to win another pageant. Nevertheless, never leave the auditorium feeling defeated. Be true to yourself," says Mary Francis Flood. Furthermore, "Knowing who you are and know that when you're faced with a mountain, you will not quit. You will keep striving until you climb over it and if you can't climb over it, you'll find a tunnel underneath, or you'll simply stay and turn this terrific mountain into a gold mine." Says San Diego pageant contestant Kathy Eidsmoe, "No matter how many times you lose, it does not get easier, and it hurts. You just have to accept it and go on to the next challenge."

A true winner helps others to be winners. There is no failure in life if we learn by the mistakes we have made. "If you do not win this pageant, your time will come," says Jane Jaffe. Anyone who made a new friend, had a good time, shared an experience of a lifetime, or learned about herself is a winner! Most importantly, to lose graciously is to be a winner. Should you win the title, look upon it as being at the right place, at the right time, with the right ingredients. "The one who's learned and grown most is the true winner," advises Barbara Kelley. "The one who uses that pageant experience to help her have a winning attitude through the rest of her life." A contestant's personal vanity, ego or determination will have a bearing on how well she will do the next time she enters. A contestant not making the semifinals or finals should try again, paying attention to all other competing contestants. If she should not place or win this next time, she should take notes of the winners performance, looking for things the winner did that others did not do.

Professional Pageant Coaches

There is a little bit of *Miss America* in everybody, if they just apply themselves to bringing it out. Being beautiful requires work! Whether or not you intend to compete on a national level, professional training is an inestimable benefit for any competitor. National competition, of course, *requires* a professional polish, and you can never possess too many competition "tips." The key to being a successful contestant is bringing out the best in yourself. Below are some profiles of pageant coaches who have helped contestants realize their dreams. Local contacts can be found by calling nearby modeling agencies or by asking former contestants for recommendations. Pageant books, publications and tapes are also treasure troves of useful pageant informations. A listing of these sources can be found in Appendix C. A listing of pointers to help you prepare for pageant competition can be found in Appendix F. A copy of this list can be used as a checklist guide.

Several outstanding Southern pageant coaches have various forms of coaching. These coaches spend hours on end training their girls for national-level competition. Some contestants meet their coaches for a few hours each week, either privately or in a class, while others move in with their coaches for 24-hour a day training. Judges are turned off by girls who appear over- coached, so there is a limit to what coaches can do. A good coach will teach the right moves so thoroughly that they become a natural part of the girl's style.

Richard Guy and Rex Holt

Richard Guy and Rex Holt acquired the franchise to the *Miss Texas USA* pageant in 1975. Since then, six of their titleholders have been crowned *Miss USA*, and all have made it to the semi-finals. Kim Tomes became the first in the string when she was crowned *Miss USA* 1977. She was followed by Laura Martinez-Herring in 1985, Christy Fichtner in 1986, Michelle Royer in 1987, Courtney Gibbs in 1988, and Gretchen Pohemus in 1989.

As soon as *Miss Texas USA* is crowned, her training begins. She moves to El Paso, occupying a third floor apartment at their headquarters. She is sent to San Francisco where a nutritionist analyzes her figure and creates an individualized diet program. She is taught exercises involving travel weights and a jump rope, since she'll be on the road and may not have the time to visit a gym. Smoking is forbidden.

Richard admits that at first she's terrified. He tells her for the next ten months to pull her tummy in and that her makeup is all wrong. He also asks her to put all her energies into her new job and to give 150 percent of herself. A girl goes to Richard and Rex, and she grows and changes.

Richard Guy and Rex Holt do not tolerate distractions such as boyfriends or parents. They interfere with their girl's growth. She doesn't need a boyfriend who thinks she's being worked to hard or who doesn't want her to grow or is jealous or resentful of her becoming more sure of herself. The arrangement with the contestant's parents is that they have given their daughter into Richard and Rex's care, and they will not call or accept calls while she is in training. They met Christy Fichtner's parents for the first time at the *Miss USA* pageant.

According to Richard Guy, if the contestant does not want to exercise, she does not have to. They do not program their titleholder to compete in pageants. They don't tell her what to do to win a beauty pageant. He feels that if he is always in control, he will have a robot, not a contestant. The only requirement for a girl, during her stay with Richard and Rex, is thinking about what she likes, what she wants and who she is. Richard tells her to buy books that interest her and to underline passages in them that she thinks are about her — anything, so he can find out who she is.

It's not looks that win a crown; it's what's inside that counts. Rex Holt and Richard Guy feel that beauty starts from within. They do not expect for a girl to be built like Raquel Welch, but she must be physically fit. This takes work, but it is necessary preparation for the swimsuit contest. Many want to know what *Miss Texas* has that others don't. It's not a "winning look" — each year the newly crowned *Miss Texas USA* looks completely different from the last. The only thing each titleholder has in common is that she has been "polished" by Richard Guy and Rex Holt.

It is not uncommon for pageant directors to force a particular look upon their contestant, fitting them into the same mold year after year. Manipulation and exploitation are what give pageants a bad name, and the success of the "Guyrex girls" demonstrates that those tactics are not only unscrupulous, they are unnecessary. A Guyrex girl doesn't fit any mold. The key to Richard Guy and Rex Holt's success is that they don't clone their girls.

Because nothing is perfect in this life, Richard Guy and Rex Holt teach their titleholder to look at the 80 percent that is positive rather than the 20 percent that's negative. As Richard Guy and Rex Holt see it, losing the crown is not a failure. They do not want a girl to feel she has to have the crown. They want her to be able to look back from the future and see that she did her best and had a great time. She should not feel like crying if she doesn't win the title.

This is, nonetheless, a rigorous training program, and not surprisingly, many pupils rebel, telling Richard and Rex that they don't like them. According to Richard, this doesn't matter; liking one another isn't in the contract. Once Richard caught Christy Fichter "slumping" at a party. "I learned over and whispered 'such it up, and keep it sucked up all night!' She did."[3] By the eve of the pageant, Christy admitted, "Guy and I were barely on speaking terms."[4]

When she started, Christy's makeup was very pink. Unfortunately, this caused people to notice her makeup rather than her. It also caused her eyes to appear smaller. At the same time her hair was short and heavily bleached. Richard Guy and Rex Holt led her to use brown tones around her eyes to open them up and to grow her hair longer and return it to its natural shade. For the *Miss USA* pageant, her state costume required a different hairstyle than did the rest of her competitions. After that initial onstage appearance, she completed the competition in an elegant French twist. Ultimately, that hairstyle was wearing the *Miss USA* crown.

Laura Martinez-Herring is of a mixed cultural heritage, that is, Spanish is the language which was spoken at home. To prepare her for the *Miss USA* pageant, Richard Guy and Rex Holt brought in a speech coach to help her dampen her Mexican accent. They required her family and friends to speak to her only in English, to accustom her to responding more quickly in that language. This was to prepare her for pageant interviews. They brought in a trainer to make her skip rope two hours a day, toning her body, and a dietitian developed a seaweed and fruit juice drink to help her lose weight. Richard Guy supplied extra motivation by calling her "tubby" at fittings.

Michelle Royer, a 21-year old part-time model, makes no bones about where the credit for her win goes, "Texas has a couple of great directors who have put their heart and soul into their pageant for 13 years. They gave me everything in the world to prepare for the pageant. Most importantly, they taught me that it was important to be myself."[5]

3   *People*, May 4, 1986
4   Ibid.
5   *Pageantry*, Spring 1987

No *Miss Texas USA* contestant enters that pageant unaware of the difficulties which await should one of them win the title. Richard Guy and Rex Holt warn all the contestants about the long road ahead. After a few months of training, *Miss Texas* begins her public appearances. These help to sharpen the social skills. Because most of her personal appearances are in the evening, they often continue until midnight. *Miss Texas* is on call twenty-four hours a day. If she tells Richard Guy that she is tired, he responds that she is too young to be tired.

Richard Guy and Rex Holt are hoping that when *Miss Texas USA* walks through their door, they will be encountering an untiring, sensible, mature, responsible person. They hope for an attractive girl who's willing to work hard, who can talk and can make others feel good. They are looking for the overall package. "She's got to sell Texas and know how to market herself."[6] To Richard Guy, beauty queens are "walking advertisements."

Richard Guy and Rex Holt recently assumed the directorship of the California *Miss USA* franchise. They hope to do the same thing there that they have done in Texas. In the 1988 *Miss USA* pageant Richard remembers, "When it was down to th two girls [*Miss Texas* and *Miss California*], I just said we can't lose. Heads or Tails!"[7]

Obviously, the formula Richard Guy and Rex Holt have been perfecting works, and each year, the legend builds. "They really have perfected the art of developing contestants for beauty pageants. They prepare them correctly. They design the gowns. They groom them. And they win," says *Miss USA* pageant spokesman Les Schecter.[8]

Mary Francis Flood

Mary Francis Flood lives in Leland, Mississippi. She had been coaching contestants for 32 years. "In order to be a good pageant coach, you must have several of the necessary qualifications," she

---

6   *The San Antonio Light*, July 27, 1983
7   *USA Today*, March 3, 1988
8   Ibid.

reports. "You must have at one point in your life been on the runway yourself, whether it be as a professional model or as a former contestant. You must care about the girl as an individual, because you are directing her and instructing her in many manners. The things that you teach, she will carry with her the rest of her life. You must have a balance in your life: mental fitness, spiritual fitness, physical fitness, and if at all possible, family fitness. You must not get any of these out of balance. I feel the qualifications I possess that make me a good coach is that I teach Christian coaching."

Mary Francis takes her clients into her home, where she teaches them the skills and techniques of becoming a beauty pageant winner. If a girl lives too far away to go home at night, she is allowed to stay with Mary Francis, often at no extra cost. Most girls are eager to learn how to enhance the talents they already have. For this she charges either a flat fee or an hourly rate. "Winners of beauty pageants don't get there on determination alone. They go into training to learn the proper techniques," says Mary. She insists that pageantry is something one learns how to do. It's a skill, like any other. "It can take months or years to gain the poise and look of a winner."

The first quality Mary Francis seeks in her contestants is a good attitude. Attitude can be an asset or it can be a detriment in preparing for pageant competition. "If a girl has a good attitude, she will be able to encounter whatever she encounters in the proper manner. If she does not have a positive attitude, I strive most of all to teach this." She also seeks humility in her clients. "We're not going to get through anything in life without humility," she says. Mary Francis also stresses being kind and thoughtful to other people. If you always remember these things, they are going to remember you by your "good manners and the good kind person that you are."

Mary Francis Flood accepts only clients over the age of twelve. she used to take in younger girls, but with the little ones eighty percent of the work is with the mother. It saddens Mary Francis when the mother is more ambitious than the child. Also, Mary Francis stresses losing gracefully, and little girls are not interested in learning about losing. Too often, all they want is the crown.

The techniques of direct eye contact is one that Mary Francis encourages her students to develop. "We handle people throughout life," says Mary. "Eye contact is part of the body language that can convey to other people the type of person that you really are. With good eye contact, you're saying, 'Hey, I feel good about myself and I know the direction that I am going in. I may not have all the answers, but with God's help, I'm going to try." We accept ourself, we believe in ourself, and we commit ourself." When a girl goes into an interview, she must have good eye contact, be relaxed, smile and have a sense of humor with her answers.

Mary Francis Flood prepares a client for the interview competition by encouraging her to know herself so that she can recognize her assets and emphasize them. Mary Francis teaches her client to listen to the news and to read the newspaper. "There are many ways to read the newspaper," notes mary Francis, "and I strive to teach them." She teaches her girls to listen intently to what the judges are saying. "If you do not listen intently," she admonishes, "you may take the wrong meaning out of the question. If you do not know the answer, then you must tell them 'I'm sorry, I do not know.'"

Many things go into preparing a Mary Francis Flood girl for the swimsuit competition. For most, it's her overall appearance that counts. "Does she have long legs? Or is her height somewhere else other than her legs?" According to Mary Francis, height is not a major factor in doing well onstage. Instead, a girl's body should be well proportioned. "A girl that is short can be made to look tall by putting her in four inch heels and teaching her to swing her legs properly. A girl can appear to be a lot taller than she really is in the way that she is groomed." According to Mary Francis, a well-toned body is essential for the swimsuit competition.

Mary Francis Flood girls study hair styling and makeup. They spend hours under a tanning machine. They work on their bodies — some resorting to the surgical restructuring of chests, noses, chins, eyes and fannies. They learn to walk, smile and do a proper full turn. They study the way to pull their knees together and hold their feet in the 10 and 12 position. They view pictures and videotapes of previous national winners. Her girls "study" pageants. They learn to say "Yes, I have, Bob," or "That's right,

Bob," when the emcee asks them a question. They learn what clothes and jewelry to wear. They polish their runway skills at a local auditorium and learn what to do with their hands. Mary Francis emphasizes that girls must be careful in their body movements. They must walk like a lady, swing their legs from the thighs, bending at the knees and walk with the legs directly in front of one another, hitting the floor with the balls of the feet.

When asked how dedicated a girl must be to compete for a title, Mary Francis Flood responds, "She must strive to win the title." When asked what are the attributes a girl needs to develop to win, she answers, "...charisma on the runway, a nice well-toned body, learning to use body language in the way you walk, in the way you stand, in the way you sit. You are conveying to the judges and to the audience that you like yourself. You have to be careful not to appear too self-confident because when you appear too self-confident, sometimes you portray arrogance. There is a fine line between arrogance and self-confidence."

In any one pageant, Mary Francis may have as many as ten girls competing for the crown. People sometimes ask if she knows who is going to win. She replies that she knows what she wants, but that that isn't necessarily the same thing that a particular panel of judges is seeking. So, no she doesn't know ahead who is going to win. She teaches each girl to be the very best that she can be. A winner will have consistently outstanding throughout the pageant. She will have had a sparkle in her eye and a genuine smile on he face — two of the hallmarks of a winner.

Kristi Addis, *Miss Mississippi Teen USA* 1987, was coached by Mary Francis Flood. After she won the *Miss Teen USA* title that year, she said, "The greatest thing Mary Francis did for me was make me feel comfortable with myself."

Barbara Kelley and "The Winning Look"

Barbara Kelley represented Virginia in the 1958 *Miss America* pageant. Today she travels across the United States, conducting "The Winning Look" motivational seminars for contestants in the *Miss America, Mrs. America*, and *Miss USA* pageants, among many others. Barbara knows what judges are seeking; she, herself, has thirty years of state level judging experience. She notes, "In the

Miss America pageant, the judges are realizing more and more that the titleholder must talk to the press and to an audience each time she appears. *Miss America* use to be thought of as an entertainer, but today she will give speeches more times than she will perform her talent."

During "The Winning Look" seminars, she emphasizes, amongst the tips to help win, that getting the most out of a pageant, whether one wins or loses is the measure of success. She shares secrets of pageant preparedness, discussing how to arrange a pageant wardrobe, handle the judges' interview questions, apply professional makeup, walk the runway and develop a winning talent and attitude. "I try to take the experience I've had both as a contestant and as a judge. Coming from these directions, I show girls how to put their best foot forward and develop the attitude of a winner — not only for pageants, but for the rest of their lives as well."

Among the areas covered in the seminar is swimsuits. It is essential in this area of competition for a girl to have a healthy body. This is defined in terms of a firm bottom, flat stomach and no cellulite to make thighs jiggle. "Maintaining your body," advises Barbara, "shows judges that you can handle responsibility and have the determination it takes to be a winner." She also teaches how to choose the right suit to flatter that body. The right suit can hide figure flaws and emphasize strong points. Barbara notes that a Virginia designer tie-dies suits to shade big hips or accent attractive breasts. Another, in South Carolina, uses the client's measurements and a computer to design a suit specifically for that client. Barbara recommends that before the pageant, contestants practice walking for thirty minutes a day for thirty days in their heels and swimsuit. This half hour should be split between walking down a hallway in front of a mirror and walking on carpeting and stairs. She also recommends an additional 30 minutes practice for thirty days before a pageant in evening gown and heels. That way, "You wear the gown rather than it wearing you — that's the real secret to a graceful presence on the runway!"

Occasionally, Barbara Kelley will advise a contestant to drop out of competition for a year, to develop the emotional and intellectual sides of her personality. She notes, "Knowing what to expect in a pageant and preparing for it is a good idea, but you can become obsessed with pageants to the point of losing your own personality."

Barbara also uses her expertise to teach retail salespeople to properly sell the best color, style and fit of competition gowns and swimsuits. She appears 25 times a year, as guest lecturer, at the apparel markets in New York, Los Angeles, Chicago, Dallas and Atlanta. She has also been the featured speaker at Production Workshops in both the *Miss America* and *Miss USA* pageant systems.

The Competitive Edge

The Competitive Edge is a nationally organized "Queen Service." It aids aspiring queens in equestrian pageantry by teaching them the elements which comprise the Personality and Appearance categories of competition. The service provides training in three packages: *The Competitive Edge News*, The Competitive Edge Seminars, and The Competitive Edge Coaching. Each of these covers wardrobing and fashion tips, cosmetic application, skin care, speech and interviewing techniques, organizational skills, and most importantly, attitude and self-confidence. "I know if they hadn't helped me, I wouldn't have done as well at nationals," one 18-year-old said. "They put the finishing edge on everything. They put me together. I was happy."[9]

Debra Fox and Teddi Bankes-Domann, both former *Miss Rodeo Kansas* queen, created this service to share their interest, knowledge, research, personal career training and personal experiences with other contestants. They hope this will allow their clients to save time and money, help them understand the theories of competition and become more confident in themselves. They have leaned that becoming a queen can be costly and time consuming if one doesn't know the "ins and outs" of competing. Teddi notes, "We highly encourage the mothers to attend the seminar with their daughters because the two must become a working team."[10] In their services, they also teach what is involved in being a public relations specialist, promoting an in-

9   *New York Times*, December 5, 1987
10   *The Competitive Edge News*

dustry, via a crown.

More Information

For more information on coaching and on coaches, see Appendix
G.

Chapter 5

The Pageant and Beyond

By now, if you are still reading this book, you have decided, "I can do that." The next, crucial step is to decide which pageant to enter. One of the factors that will help you determine the right pageant for you is the time commitment, both during the pageant and in the event that you win. If you have to coordinate a school or work schedule with pageant obligations, you may cause yourself a severe dilemma by not knowing all the participation requirements ahead of time. You may find it more practical to limit your pageant participation to the summer months, but if you are selected queen, you should be prepared to sacrifice your time and energy to meet the demands of the title.

Know the Pageant Schedule

You should also know the pageant schedule, so that you can prepare your wardrobe. If pool parties are scheduled, you will need extra swimsuits. You will need to know how densely packed the schedule is. How many extra outfits will you have to pack, to be prepared for unexpected schedule changes. Will the pageant you are contemplating include an opening production number? If so, how many songs will you have to memorize and what costumes will you need to assemble for the number? In any case, you will want to bring comfortable shoes to wear during rehearsals. You will need to look your best at all times. You never know when the media will be around.

Winning a pageant is not as glamorous as many people think.

For many national queens, the year they spend representing their title is like getting a Ph.D. in human relations. It teaches them a lot about people, about adjusting, about growing. The road which lies ahead for national titleholders is a long and hard one. There are many displeasures according to *Becoming a Beauty Queen*. They include catching 4:00 a.m. flights, changing clothes in airplane lavatories, packing and unpacking suitcases, doing laundry in the bathtub, and returning to hotel rooms late at night only to get up for early morning appearances.

Know the Rules

Another consideration is whether you will be able to enter other pageants while you hold the title for which you are considering competing. This may not seem important now; but in the event you do win, your title may be forfeited if you continue entering other pageants. Know all the rules and regulations before you enter a pageant.

Entering a local, well-established pageant is often ideal for the first-time contender. Because no two pageants are the same, you will want to find out all the facts beforehand, so you can choose the right one. You should establish exactly what your financial and contractual obligations will be. You should know the scholastic and time requirements as well as scoring procedures and appearances the titleholder will be expected to make *before* you enter. To ensure that you ask all the right questions, — and remember the answers, — create a list of questions. When you are seeking the right pageant, have your list handy and ask all your questions. Karyl Gammon warns, "Do not be afraid to ask the director for names and phone numbers of one or two past winners as a reference." She also suggests that you watch the competition, noting its professionalism. After the pageant, talk with some of the mothers and contestants for feedback. Karyl's daughter Brandi Gammon makes her pageant choices based on her long-term goal. She advises, "If your goal is to be *Miss America* or *Miss USA*, you enter local pageants tailored to either system." Kelli Lee, *Miss South Texas Teen* 1985, makes her pageant choice by considering the prizes offered, the areas of competition and what opportunities are likely to arise from such exposure.

Know the Prize Structure

Know what the prize structure is. Will the cash "scholarships" be limited for educational use only? In the event that you cannot use a particular prize, such as a modeling scholarship, is it transferable? Will the prize package offered be immediately available to the winner? Obtain the address of last year's reigning queen and find out if all promised prizes were received promptly. Another sign of the professionalism of a pageant system is taking the time to interview prospective contestants, eliminating negative contestants in the preliminary stages.

Advertised Pageants

Most pageant directors advertise their pageants in the Lifestyle, Fashion, and miscellaneous sections of the local newspaper. Also look in high school and college newspapers for pageant advertisements. Modeling schools are usually informed about pageants, so you might want to call a few. For the most part girls receive applications in the mail. Ask friends who have competed in pageants both for their recommendations as to which pageants to enter and to have them pass your name on to pageant directors to be included on pageant mailing lists. Be aware that, as Bob Marshall, editor of the *Pageant Review*, says, "A legitimate competition lives up to its advertising." At the first sign that a pageant is not living up to its promises, investigate promptly and protect your interests.

Magazine Contests

Many magazines offer opportunities for women to win valuable prizes by entering their contests. For example, every year 'TEEN magazine sponsors *'TEEN's Great Model Search*. Sixteen regional semifinalists are chosen monthly to advance to the next level of competition. Entries should include one headshot and one full-length photograph. Make sure your photos are in focus and that your name is on the back of each photo. On a sheet of paper write your name, address, city, state, zip code, age, date of birth, home phone, height, weight, measurements, and hobbies/special interests. Also include $1 by check or money order, payable to 'TEEN, to cover handling costs. Attach a note, signed by your parents or guardian, stating "If I am chosen as a finalist, I agree to the use of my name and/or likeness in *'TEEN* magazine and its associated companies. If I am chosen as a winner, I agree to enter a one-year exclusive modeling contract with The Gillette Company in the health and beauty aids company." Send all information to: *Great Model Search, 'TEEN* Magazine, P.O. Box 69940, Los Angeles, CA 90069.

Seventeen Magazine holds a *Cover Model* contest, annually. The contest is open to young women between the ages of 13 and 21. Entry forms can be picked up at the *Seventeen's Cover Model* contest headquarters nearest you. To find its location, look in the March issue of *Seventeen*, or write to Triangle Communications, Inc., 850 Third Avenue, New York, NY 10022.

Know the Expenses Involved

Know, ahead of time, all the expenses involved in participating. What financial obligations are required of contestants? Pageant directors have been known to register girls into their pageants, only to tell them later that other purchases were mandatory. For example, you pay your sponsorship fee and *then* the director tells you that you are also required to purchase pageant t-shirts to wear as part of the production number, or that it is mandatory for you to sell advertisements in the pageant program booklet or out-of-town attendance tickets. All financial obligations should be spelled out in writing, with the notation "and no other" before you sign a participation contract or entry form.

You should also have a firm grasp of which expenses the pageant will bear and which you will be undertaking for yourself. Most pageants require girls to purchase their own evening gowns, but some will provide competition swimsuits for their contestants or arrange for a group purchase discount. Once, I judged a state pageant in which one contestant arrived at the pageant location with no competition outfits. She had thought that the sponsorship fee covered these items and that they would be made available to her at the state pageant. Also make sure that you know what expenses you, personally will be asked to bear if you are the titleholder. It would be heartbreaking to have to forfeit your title because you could not afford to fulfill the obligations! At a minimum, the pageant organization should cover the titleholder and chaperon's traveling expenses, including meals, lodging and mileage.

Pageant Facilities and Sleeping Accommodations

Pageant facilities and sleeping accommodations are another aspect of pageant participation that should hold no surprises for the contestants. Accommodations can run from private hotel rooms to college dorms. Do you, as the contestant, pay for your accommodations, or are they included in the fee structure? One Texas pageant director arranges for local town families to host a contestant or two in their homes over the entire pageant weekend. These host families will support the contestant for the entire weekend, feeding her two or three meals a day and giving her emotional support. For most contestants, these hosts become second families, making lasting friendships.

Areas of Competition

Various pageants include different areas of competition, ranging from sportswear, aerobic wear, and western wear to leadership, essays, and community involvement. Many teen pageants stress scholastic achievement. In fact, many require contestants to take a written test that covers academic subjects. In the *Dream Girl USA* pageant, one area of competition is Body Tone. In this competition, girls are judged on their physical fitness and body form in aerobics wear. In the *San Antonio Stock Show and Rodeo Queen* pageant, contestants are expected to demonstrate their horsemanship abilities. Horsemanship is generally broken into several areas: Horsemanship, Mount and Dismount, Position of hands, feet, and seat, Appearance on horseback, Intelligence, Conversational ability, Rodeo knowledge, Knowledge of tack, Knowledge of horse care, and Involvement in a Rodeo Association.

Many pageants include community involvement as an area of competition. In this arena, girls are expected to perform a number of volunteer hours with a community or national organization. Many times a contestant is uncertain what type of community work to do. If this should happen to you, consider teaching an illiterate person to read. Contact the Coalition for Literacy Hotline at 1-800-228-8813 for information. For other ideas write to Volunteers Under 30, P.O. Box 1987, Denver, CO 80201.

Know the Scoring System

Know what scoring system will be used to judge the pageant you are entering. "Don't set yourself up for an unwelcome surprise," notes Karen Kemple. Some pageants give equal value to all areas of competition while others give more weight to some areas. Some pageants retain preliminary scores, or some of them, while others have semifinalists compete from scratch.

Know the Composition of the Judges Panel

In this same vein, you should know what type of people have been selected to judge the pageant. Will they be politically affiliated people? Will they have a strong public relations background, be associated with a beauty magazine, a fashion consultant, a fashion photographer, a former beauty queen, an out-of-state pageant director or a modeling instructor? Will the panel be half male, half female? The answers to these questions can help you find the right pageant. Your pageant director may refuse to give you the names of the judging panel, but she should be able to tell you how they qualify.

Contractual Obligations

Most pageants require contestants to sign a contract giving the pageant exclusive rights to product endorsement and personal appearances throughout a titleholder's reign. Most contracts also include a release stating that contestants will not hold the pageant responsible in the event of an injury during pageant activities. Some contracts also stipulate that titleholders cannot participate in other pageants during her reign. Contestants may be required to sign a model's release form before they appear in publicity photo shoots. Take the time to read and understand any contract you are asked to sign — before you sign it. If possible, have an attorney review any contract you are contemplating signing.

Unscrupulous Promoters

Unscrupulous pageant promoters have been known to collect sponsorship fees and flee without contacting contestants. Contestants then show up at the pageant location to find the pageant was never scheduled to take place. Advises Karen Kemple, "Before you sign up with a pageant, call the Better Business Bureau and the Chamber of Commerce of the city in which the pageant is headquartered. See if complaints have been filed against the pageant." Call the location at which the pageant is to take place. Find out if the pageant has paid in full or placed a deposit to secure the rental. If a deposit has not been made, it's time to wonder about the pageant.

Sponsorship Fees

Most pageants require contestants to pay a sponsorship fee before participation. It is important that you and your sponsors understand the nature of sponsorship fees. This payment, sometimes called an entry fee or sub-sponsorship fee, is a flat fee assessed by the pageant director to each contestant entering the contest. It covers part of the pageant production costs, including advertising, auditorium rental, lighting, sound, hired assistants, printing costs, etc. For example, the 1988 *Miss Texas USA* pageant took in $317,000 from ad and ticket sales as well as from contestant entry fees, and spent $305,000. Their television costs alone were $82,000.

The sponsorship fee is raised by contributions from individuals and businesses. Whoever supports a contestant by paying any part of the sponsorship fee qualifies as a sponsor. Contestants who live in remote areas or who do not have time to secure outside sponsorship may sponsor themselves. Those who are self-sponsored may include the name of their favorite charity in their sponsor listing. Some girls, unable for one reason or another, to raise the entry fee, have been known to seek employment to earn the money.

Finding Sponsors

Realizing that the sponsorship fee is to finance the production costs of the pageant rather than to provide you with a nest egg makes it easier for you to represent the proposal to prospective sponsors. It also makes businesses and individuals more receptive to representing you. Some pageants limit the number of sponsors to no more than five or six per girl. Others will allow as many as needed to come up with the required fee. Know the requirements of your pageant before you begin soliciting support.

Recognize that businesses plan their budgets far in advance. You need to give them time to include the pageant in their planning. Franchised companies are more difficult to obtain and should be approached months before a pageant. In the meantime, while you await the franchise's response, contact local merchants. It is wise to solicit lots of prospective sponsors and select carefully from the ones who agree to sponsorship. Get a head start by making a list of the people you know from the business world. Put businesses you patronize frequently, like your hairdresser, your manicurist, the dry cleaner, doctor and diet center, at the top of your list. If you are employed, make contacts within your company. If you run out of contacts, make cold calls on businesses in your community. Meet by appointment with the advertising manager, business manager or firm owner, and have your request well-prepared before the meeting. Remember that sponsorship fees are tax decuctible for the sponsor, and make that part of your pitch.

Approach your town newspaper to sponsor you with ad space. This allows you more leverage when structuring sponsorship support. For example, say you are limited to securing no more than five sponsors for your pageant entry fee. You may secure your total fee within that amount and you may not. With the sponsored ad space from your town paper, you can list your pageant sponsors as well as the people and businesses who have donated their time and merchandise in preparation for your pageant. Besides, local merchants might prefer seeing their company name in a local medium. The benefit of this situation is that you can list more than five sponsors in a advertisement that was *sponsored* by your town paper! This makes securing local sponsorship support much easier.

New businesses flourish daily, and you can find the names of these new businesses to contact for sponsorship support. For instance, in San Diego, you can purchase a listing of new businesses and their addresses from the City Hall. For a nominal fee, you will receive a single listing of new businesses. These companies tend to be receptive to advertising and promotion. So, contacting them is smart.

Ideas for raising sponsorship fee are limited only by the limits of creativity. Successful projects have included garage sales, bake sales, neighborhood collections, etc. The Texas economy being depressed, it was not easy for Kelli Lee to secure her $1,100 entry fee for the *Miss Texas USA* pageant. She raised money by trading her services as a spokesmodel for one year's worth of appearances. Another contestant raffled off a stuffed teddy bear. You should, of course, demonstrate your responsibility and resourcefulness by earning your sponsorship fee, rather than merely asking for the money.

Do not be disappointed if a local business manager seems interested in sponsoring you, but then decides it will not benefit the company. Not all businesses will support pageants.

Sometimes contestants are uncertain when to collect the money from their sponsors. Obtain the money as soon as the business has made a verbal commitment. Some businesses will write out a check on the spot, others will prefer to mail the fee to the pageant headquarters. If you receive the money yourself, be prepared to issue a receipt at the same time that you take possession of the money. Make sure you know how and when your sponsorship fee is due. Are you to turn it in as soon as you collect it? Are you to turn it in as you gather it, or all at once. Some pageants have installment plans. Be sure you know the pageant structure of your pageant.

Incentives

Some pageants encourage their contestant to be go-getters, allowing them to keep anything received above the required entry fee. The extra money, then, can pay for costs such as competition outfits and additional outfits needed for scheduled pageant events. Others pageants offer participation incentives. Instead of tying the incentive to sponsorship, they tie it to bringing in other contestants. A pageant director may offer a 25% cash refund for contestants who get one friend to register, 50% for two and free entry for three or more. This means that if you get three friends to enter the pageant, you will be allowed to enter for free. If your pageant does not offer this incentive, ask them to make an exception.

A Helpful Support Guide

I have devised a helpful support guide to assist you with your presentation to your prospective sponsors. Use it as a guide, memorizing it and practicing until it sounds completely natural. While many contestants secure sponsors over the phone, it is best to make your contacts in person. Let's face it, it is easier to say "NO" over the phone than it is in person. See Appendix A for the contestant support guide.

Your Entry Package

Now, having found the right pageant, investigated it thoroughly, and planned how you will raise the sponsorship fee, it is time to get your entry package in order.

The Entry Form

The entry form is the first official step in entering a pageant, and it is important that you understand how significant that step is. The application communicates your character to the judges. It also serves as the source of interview questions, onstage questions, and emcee information. Be sure yours sounds interesting and professional. Write on your application as you would a job résumé — very carefully. Be prepared to explain in detail every fact you have listed. In the same vein, list the most important and interesting items first in each category. These first items will be more noticeable when the entry is skimmed hurriedly.

Prior to winning the 1980 *Miss America* crown, Cheryl Prewitt-Salem prepared for the pageant under the watchful eye of Pat and Briggs Hopson. With a sharp eye for detail Briggs took special care to tailor Cheryl's application to her best advantage. During a mock interview Briggs questioned Cheryl with her application in hand:

"Hm-m," he said, adjusting his glasses as he studied the sheet. "I see here you've listed cooking as one of your hobbies. Tell me, how do you make a crepe?"

"A crepe?" I said. "Gosh, I don't know."

"Soufflé?" I repeated. "I'm afraid I don't know that, either."

"Well," said Briggs, regarding me curiously, "what kind of foods can you cook?"

"Oh," I said, "you know — things like black-eyed peas, country-fried chicken, homemade corn bread."

"Ah-h," grinned Briggs, "you mean *southern* cooking."[1]

Make several copies of the blank application. Fill out the first copy in pencil, reading it over several times and checking your spelling, grammar and sentence structure. Barbara Kelley suggests that you have several people — family, friends, and a business acquaintance — go over your application and make suggestions. If at all possible, type the final copy or have it typed. If this is just not possible, print your information very neatly and clearly.

Make sure that the information on your entry form is as accurate and honest as possible. If you are not certain about a particular item, leave it blank and complete it later. Make you entry form as interesting as possible, being proud of your accomplishments. Mary Francis Flood notes, "Girls should assess and emphasize their strengths, but not try to be someone they're not." Give each item careful thought when filling out your application. Karen Kemple suggest that you include some "teasers" to pique the interest of the judges. If a second page is necessary, type "see attachment" or "continued on back" on the front side of your application.

Do not embroider the facts. If you are not 115 pounds, don't claim it. If you see future changes in items such as your weight, leave that space blank until a week or so before before the pageant to accommodate the success of your training program. Simply call up the director and ask that your current weight be added to the application. This applies to other changes as well, including your grade-point average, or winning a position in a class election. If you do have a last minute change or addition, most pageant directors will permit you to submit a revised copy. Be sure you

1   Cheryl Prewitt-Salem, *A Bright Shining Place*, Praise Books, 1981, p. 231.

keep a copy of your application — both for your files and to aid your preparation.

Birth Certificates, Transcripts, and Black and White Photographs

You may need to produce a copy of your birth certificate and/or a transcript of your grades. You should have certified copies of these in your pageant preparation file. After you have retained your sponsors, the next step is to determine whether the pageant will be including photos in the program booklet. If they are, you should arrange for a flattering portrait. It could provide the judges' first glimpse of how you look. Make sure the photograph looks like you. If you submit photos which are too touched up, the judges may be disappointed when they meet you. Similarly, do not submit a photo in which your color appears different or your style is drastically different.

Remember that black and white photographs give sharp reproductions whereas color photographs tend to give dark and grainy ones. If your photograph has too much background, the reproduction will not be clear. Similarly, avoid over-the- shoulder sexy looks. Your photograph should show a happy, pleasing face. The makeup to produce this result is different from that for color photography. When preparing for a black and white shoot, it is important to think of your makeup in terms of tones instead of colors. It doesn't matter if your eyeshadow is blue or purple. What matters is if it is deep or pale blue. With black and white film, all colors photograph as black, white or shades of gray. Consequently, it is important that you create shadows of illusion by having contrast in the proper areas.

Competition Night

The final area of pageant preparation, is mentally rehearsing the events of the evening competition. The more you know about the mechanics of the judges and crowning, the more at ease you will be, and as stressed above, the more confident you will appear — the more like a winner.

Judging

Judges generally cast a total of 3 ballots during the preliminary part of the competition. Most commonly, these are one each for the interview, the swimsuit, and the evening gown. Scoring in most pageants is based on a scale of 1 to 10 in each area of competition. After the auditor has tabulated all the scores, the ten contestants with the highest scores will be named semifinalists.

The Pop-Question

At this point, the master of ceremonies will generally interview each semifinalist onstage, usually by asking a pop-question. These questions test each girl's ability to think on her feet. In the 1969 *Maid of Cotton* pageant, Cathy Muirhead was asked, "What would you do if you were at a football game, and your wig fell off?" Cathy responded, "I'd jump up and holler 'Somebody stomp on that thing!'"[2] The wire accounts of Cathy's answer appeared in papers across the nation. One radio station awarded her a certificate for having created the top news story of the week.

The *Miss USA* pageant has a different approach to the finalist pop-question. They ask that contestants bring snapshots of various time periods in their lives. These could include their first birthday party, performing in an elementary school play, their prom night, etc. The host selects a picture and asks the finalist to talk about it. This is a sure way of bringing out her personality. In the 1988 *U.S. Man of the Year* pageant, finalists were asked questions by the audience, like on the Phil Donahue or Oprah Winfrey shows.

Finalists and Tie-Breakers

From the semifinalists, five finalists are selected. The judges determine these by ranking them in order of preference on a final ballot. In the event of a tie, each judge receives a tie-breaker ballot containing the names of the tied finalists, but not their tying positions. The judges mark their preference and return their ballot to the auditor. When completed, signed and audited, the ballot with the final decision is ready for the master of ceremonies.

2   *Public Relations Journal,* May 1969

No one in the audience, on the staff or judging panel knows the outcome of the tabulation until it is announced from the stage.

Your Scores

After the pageant, ask your pageant director if you can retain a copy of your scores. I like to assure contestants that my pageant is fair by providing the computer tabulation in front of the audience as well as giving the contestant their scores after the pageant.

Once you have been crowned with the title, your job has, literally, just begun. Before the whirl becomes overwhelming, send thank you notes, but not flowers, to the judges to demonstrate your appreciation. This assures them that they have chosen the right girl for the title.

Additional Competitions

It is advantageous for both you and your pageant director if you advance to another program. By advancing titleholders, pageant directors build the importance of their pageant. In the 1987 pageant, 26 of the 103 contestants had competed in a local pageant to win the chance to vie for the *Miss Texas USA* title. The other 77 had entered as at-large candidates, referred by area directors or friends.

If your pageant enters you in a magazine contest or advances you to another pageant, or if you decide to enter another contest on your own, make sure that the entry contract and the winner's responsibilities are not in conflict with the contract you have with the pageant you currently represent. This warning also applies to the photographers and modeling agencies that will offer you photographs and modeling courses that you may not need. Check out these individuals before you follow up on their offers, and "carefully read and understand their contacts, so that you don't end up with contractual conflicts," advises Karen Kemple.

If your pageant does not advance to another level of competition, ask your director to help you design an entry package for one of the magazine contests listed above and to write to any of the pageants listed in Appendix H for contestant information. Most pageants will be glad to have you as part of their pageant.

Your Manager and Chaperon

Besides additional competitions, a year of excitement awaits you as titleholder. There will be fun-filled events promoting goodwill for your pageant and sponsors. A manager will help make your reign a pleasant and memorable one. Your manager will ensure that you take advantage of your title in the best ways possible. This person will be responsible for arranging your appearances and for maintaining your well being. She may also act as a chaperon. A competent, adult, *female*, must accompany you during any promotional appearance. This will lessen the chance that an unscrupulous person can take advantage of you. Chaperons can also serve as an intermediary between you, as queen, and the public. She can arrange last minute details and can terminate your appearance, leaving you free to be 100% gracious to the public.

Promoting Your Title

A true winner is eager to work to promote the title she has won. She "does not merely take home the prizes, put them in the closet and go on," says Kelli Lee. "A true winner lives up to the expectations of the judges and the promoters. A true winner works in the area of community service as well as in the area of promotion. A true winner makes everyone proud of her, and she can be proud of herself." She makes her year a sharing time.

Business Cards

Your reign will not only be personally and financially rewarding, it will also be a learning experience. Remember to take advantage of these opportunities for growth. Most titleholders fade from the limelight as quickly as they gain the stage. Pageants should be viewed as one step in a life of striving, not as the end of the path. Use your year of appearances as an opportunity to make contacts and set up a career. To facilitate making contacts, have business cards ready. This demonstrates your professionalism. If you do not want to include your home address or phone number on your titleholder business cards, your manager or pageant director may allow you to substitute theirs. You may not do this, however, without their written permission.

You should have your business cards ready whenever you make a promotional appearance. For example, for years reigning queens have presided over ribbon cutting ceremonies and the dedications of new businesses. Small towns, particularly, relish these occasions. The ribbon cuttings, especially when covered by the news media, provide titleholders with tremendous exposure and opportunities to make contacts. In anticipation of your public appearances, you should practice your speaking techniques. It is said that Christy Fichtner, *Miss Texas USA* 1986, had difficulty with public speaking, in the beginning. Richard Guy and Rex Holt, directors of that pageant, worked with her, preparing a 45-minute speech for her to deliver. After she perfected that, she was fine speaking to large audiences.

Voice-Over Workshops

Another opportunity for growth is the voice-over workshop. The skills developed can aid in public speaking appearances, particularly if you are interested in pursuing a career in the broadcast field. Voice-over workshops focus on cold reading, phrasing, voice exercises, and copy interpretation. They also teach techniques of voice control. This training can be put to use in radio and television interviews promoting your pageant and its promoters.

Appearances, Autograph Signings, and Interviews

A queen's appearance is often welcomed on television shows. Some stations may even allow her to perform her talent. Young girls admire beauty queens and believe in Cinderella fantasy, making a children's show a natural. If you do this, be prepared. One little girl asked Kylene Barker Brandon, *Miss America* 1979, if she lived in a castle! The winner of the *Hal Jackson's Talented Teen*, appears on the syndicated TV show "Don Cornelius's Soul Train International." Titleholders can also appear on the local Public Broadcasting Television membership drive. While representing my title in the *Miss Buccaneer Days* pageant, I appeared as a guest host for an auction show on the public broadcast television network, as well as making a guest appearance on one network affiliate's evening news.

As queen, you will also be asked to grant radio interviews. Before you appear, you should listen to the radio show to get an advance idea of the interviewer's style. You should learn to take control of the interview, choosing the areas you wish to discuss as well as deflecting offensive questions gracefully. Finally, you should pay attention to the image your voice projects. On radio, that is all the audience will "see," and it represents both you and your pageant.

As with a radio interview, know and clear the topic of all print interviews before you agree to them. Your manager should act as your front man for these appointments, making sure you know the subject of the interview, which publication will print it, and what questions will be asked.

As titleholder, you should expect to ride on floats in town parades and attend autograph signings. At pageant functions, you should always respond graciously and affirmatively to requests for your autograph. A beauty Queen is the ideal Miss of the public an should be flattered that the public wants her autograph.

There is no question that autograph signings can get tedious and hectic. You will be rudely pushed and shoved, as the public competes for your autograph. This is no excuse for you to drop into the fray. Remain on your pedestal and graciously accede to each request — no matter how rudely presented. Debra Sue Maffett, *Miss America* 1983, was asked to sign 4,000 autographs in a single day. It raised a blister on her hand. It goes with the territory, and you should be prepared.

Inexpensive, lithograph pictures are ideal to use for autograph signings. Provide your pageant director with a master picture, from which the lithographs will be make, that is sharp in contrast and has enough white space to provide for the autographs.

Fashion Shows, Commentary, and Judging

Department stores often have in-store fashion shows. Your pageant director may arrange for you to be included in these, either as a model or as a commentator. Similarly, you may be asked to provide commentary at special functions, including other pageants, appear at "Key to the City" presentations, and/or judge other pageants. You should never decline the opportunity to judge a pageant. It will allow you to see contestants from a different perspective — that of the judges. You will learn how hard judging is, and you can apply this knowledge to future pageant competitions.

The Farewell Speech

In addition to the speaking engagements you will encounter during your reign, you will probably have to make a farewell speech at next year's pageant, before you relinquish your crown. Your farewell speech may have to be delivered "live" or it may be taped. Your farewell speech should tell about how the pageant has helped you achieve your immediate goals and how it might help you in your future endeavors. You should be prepared to write and to deliver this speech at the pageant, but you should also be aware that this speech may be written for you. In the latter case, be prepared to suggest some points that you would like to see included, and set aside enough time that you can practice your delivery until it sounds as though you wrote it yourself.

You and the Pageant Staff

Every pageant staff wants a queen who is willing and cooperative. They also want her to become as much a part of the staff as possible, particularly when it is time to recruit contestants for next year's competition. Do your best to integrate yourself into the staff. Do what is asked of you with a smile and appreciate the opportunities this staff is providing for you. The more important you help your title to become, the greater the honor it will be to have held it.

Becoming a Pageant Director

Once you can no longer participate in pageants, you should consider becoming a pageant director. Undoubtedly, you found that pageants were fun, rewarding, and learning experiences. Staying in the path of pageantry, then, becomes natural, and directing pageants is the way. Combine the positive moments of your pageant experiences into one pageant to make it exciting for a new generation of contestants. Like me, you can make your yearly goal that of continuously upgrading your pageants. You may think you are too young to become a pageant director. I was 23. An advantage to directing pageants while you are young is that you can more easily relate to your contestants. For example, it is likely you will like the same music that they do.

Becoming a pageant director is not as difficult as you may think. There are many legal details you must handle, but with the help in my book *Producing Beauty Pageants: A Director's Guide,* you can learn everything you need to know. This book covers all aspects of becoming a pageant director, from creating and registering your company name and pageant title to finding pageant sponsors and recruiting contestants. For information on ordering this book, see the order form at the end of this book.

Appendix A

Contestant Support Guide

Hello, I am_____. I have been selected to participate in the Miss _____ Pageant, where scholarships, prizes, and awards will be presented. If I win, I will be eligible to participate in the upcoming Miss _____ pageant (if your pageant leads on). I need sponsors such as you to help me so that I can accept this honor. The sponsor fee is $____. If you cannot sponsor the entire amount, any part would be appreciated. In return for your sponsorship, you will receive promotion throughout this pageant. Your company name will appear in our program and will be announced as I appear on stage. I will be happy to assist you in any way with promotional work, such as ribbon cuttings, autograph signings, drawings, etc. I will do my best to represent you as my sponsor in this pageant. I want to thank you for allowing me the time to talk with you. (Now show them the sponsorship information form.)

Appendix B

Typical Pageant Questions

- What would you do to improve your community's image?
- What constitutes true beauty?
- What is one quality that animals have that you would like to have and why?
- Do you think that community awareness is good? Why or why not?
- Do you feel that individuality is a asset or liability?
- Who is the one person that has inspired you the most in your life?
- What does friendship mean to you?
- If you could change places with someone well known for one day, who would it be and why?
- Who do you admire most in life and why?
- How forgiving are you when your friends let you down?
- Do you feel being a wife and mother will be a sufficient challenge for you or do you want a business career and why?
- Can you be counted on to do what you say you'll do?
- If you were a parent, what one value would you teach your child?
- What is your definition of beauty?
- What do you feel all well-known successful women have in common?
- What is the greatest challenge young people face today?
- A good listener or a good talker — which one is most important?
- What do you want out of life today, tomorrow, and in the future?
- Are young people more sophisticated in today's generation?
- What is your idea of a perfect man?
- What kind of person would you describe yourself as?
- If you could change something about yourself, what would it be?
- Tell of an experience that has been educational to you and why.
- Tell of a book you've read that has influenced your life and why.
- Who is the most important person to you and why?
- What advice would you give a friend entering a beauty pageant?
- How do you handle peer pressure?
- Do you think higher education is important today and why?
- In what ways would being Miss ... help you?
- What is your definition of the word "success."
- If you could contribute one thing to this world, what would it be?
- How does competition help you as a person?

- Why did you enter the Miss ... pageant?
- What do you like most about yourself?
- As a child, what was your favorite game and why?
- What attributes do you think of when you consider a teenage girl?
- If you could travel anywhere in the world, where would it be?
- Which occupation do you feel would be the most rewarding for you and why?
- What is your greatest fear?
- How would you describe your own personality?
- Which subject in school do you find most interesting and why?
- If you could date anyone in the world, who would it be and why?
- If you notice a self-destructive behavior pattern in a friend who is clearly unaware of it, would you point it out, even if it may cost you the friendship?
- What activities are you involved in at your school?
- What does friendship mean to you?
- What do you feel are your accomplishments and what are your ambitions in life?
- What qualities do you have that makes you feel that you could represent the Miss ... pageant?
- What do you plan to major in at college?
- What goals do you plan to achieve while in high school?
- How do your interests affect your lifestyle?
- What is the top asset that you feel someone needs to make it in life?
- What are your goals for the next year and for the next five years?
- What benefits do you plan to achieve from this pageant?
- What are some of the advantages of living in (city)?
- Complete this sentence: Love is _____.
- What would constitute a "perfect" evening for you?
- If you could wake up tomorrow having gained one ability or quality, what would it be?
- What is your most treasured memory?
- How do you react when people sing "Happy Birthday" to you in a public place?
- For what in your life do you feel most grateful?
- Do you feel that advice from older people carries a special weight because of their greater experience?
- Do you find it so hard to say "No" that you do favors that you really do not want to do?
- What do you value most in a relationship?
- Is there any question that you would like to ask any of the judges?
- What one word describes yourself?
- If you were about to get married and then you found out that your husband-to-be was on drugs, what would you do? Would you drop him, would you continue the wedding plans, or would you postpone the wedding and try to help him?
- What is the best gift you've received and why?

- Socrates said "know thyself." Name your best quality. Name your worst.
- In this decade, what do you think the prime ingredients are for a woman to succeed in this world?
- Tell when an act of friendship made the difference.
- How forgiving are you when your friends let you down?
- Can you be counted on to do what you say you'll do?
- What does it mean that "no man is an island"?
- What is femininity?
- Define a "lady"
- What does being an American mean to you?
- What advice would you give to a younger brother or sister?
- What is your philosophy of life?
- Describe your personality in three adjectives.
- What is your opinion of beauty pageants?
- Where do you see yourself in 10 years?
- If you had your chance of living one fantasy in your life, what would it be?
- What is a pageant?
- What is the difference between confidence and conceit?
- If you win, are you ready to handle what lies ahead?
- Are you superstitious?
- Does being mentally prepared for your talent presentation have anything to do with being physically prepared?
- If you could change one thing about your school system, what would it be?
- What do you feel is the biggest problem between parents and children today?
- What are the positive things you see about yourself that you would like everyone to know?
- Do you believe there is a generation gap?
- What have you learned most from preparing for this pageant?
- What qualities do you consider to make a really good teacher?
- What is your major and why did you select it?
- How do you perceive the role and responsibilities of a beauty queen?
- What makes your city special?
- What school activities are you involved in?
- If you could add a course to your school's present curriculum, what would it be?
- If you could choose to have any talent, what would it be?
- If you could be any age, what age would you be and why?
- How do you feel about teen suicide?
- Give an event, positive or negative, that has influenced your life.
- Who do you consider to be the most influential young people of today?
- How important are your goals to you?

- What attributes make up an ideal beauty queen?
- What is the most pressing problems that very young people or very old people face today?
- What makes you angry?
- What makes you least proud of your generation?
- What would you say if you were able to write your own caption in your yearbook?
- How would you describe your ideal vacation?
- What special thing would you like to accomplish in your life other than marriage or a career?
- What makes a good leader? Do you feel you are one?
- Which is more important, to be liked or respected?
- Do you have an alternative career goal in the event your immediate career plans do not work out as planned?
- How would you like to be remembered?
- What other century (past of future) would you like to live in and why?
- What is your biggest fantasy?
- What one person in past history do you admire most and why?
- If you were to win this title, how would you use this experience?
- What do you hope to be doing five years from now?
- Would you like to compete again even if you do not win this pageant?
- What would you do if you tripped onstage in front of a large audience?
- How do you feel about invasion of privacy should you become Miss...?
- If you could change one thing in our judicial system, what would it be?
- What country, other than the U.S., would you like to live in and why?
- What has been the most difficult thing about this pageant for you?
- What is your favorite book and why?
- Who do you consider to be the most influential women of today?
- What are your best or strongest traits?
- What has been the proudest moment of your life?
- What is your most rewarding moment in life?
- What do you treasure most about your life?
- What is the funniest thing that has ever happened to you?
- What motivates you and why?
- What is the most interesting thing about yourself?
- What are your worst habits?
- Do you feel participating in a pageant teaches one determination and responsibility?
- If you woke up tomorrow and discovered you were a boy, how would your life be different?
- What do you think was the most important discovery during the past quarter century?

- What woman in public life do you think the most of and why?
- If you could give advice to a girl who was just 4'8" tall, what would it be?
- How do you feel about the "recreational use" of drugs?
- How did you prepare for this pageant?
- Do you really want to be Miss...? Why?
- What does this pageant mean to you?
- What is the best advice you've ever received?
- What kind of girl would you describe yourself as?
- "Women's Liberation" — What does it mean to you?
- What achievement would you most want to be remembered for and why?
- If you had a choice of living anywhere in the world, where would it be?
- What is the greatest problem the world faces today?
- Should women be allowed in the armed forces?
- Should women be allowed to compete in "traditionally male" sports?
- Define patriotism.
- What is your best method of relaxation?
- When you pick up a newspaper, what is the first thing you read? The last thing?
- What do you think you will be doing ten years from now?
- If chosen as the queen, what can you contribute to the pageant organization?
- What do you consider to be the role of a beauty queen?
- If your house was on fire, what one thing would you grab on the way out?
- Looking back over this year, what accomplishment has given you the most pleasure?
- Do you feel that pageants sexually exploit women?
- Why did you select the outfit you are wearing?
- How do you feel a Miss... should dress?
- Should a woman put off child-bearing to advance her career?
- What are the most important characteristics a crownholder should possess?
- You're a grown person now. You have just been told you have been adopted. How would you react?
- What do you feel is the most important aspect of competition?
- What characteristic do you least like about yourself?
- As a role model as Miss ..., you are expected to set an example. What one example would you set?
- What is your viewpoint on balancing career and family?
- If there is one message you could share with someone special, what would it be, and to whom?
- What is the most interesting aspect of your state and why would someone want to visit it?

What do you think of the way TV covers the news?

- Do you believe in Mr. Right?
- How do you view the need for education in today's society?
- When you raise your children, will you be a strict parent or a permissive parent and why?
- Who, in your opinion, is a great man? Woman?
- Do you believe in love at first sight?
- Do you think a lady should propose to a man in our modern age?
- To your mind what is the greatest invention in the history of the world?
- What do you expect to get out of this pageant?
- Define "strength."
- Define "loyalty."
- What qualities do you think the perfect male companion should have?
- Why do you think you would make a good Miss...?
- Define sex appeal.
- Do you have any conflicting views on pageants?
- Tell me the proper way to eat lobster.
- What do you consider your biggest accomplishment to date?
- What have pageants done for you?
- If you could visit one state in the United States, which state would you choose?
- What do you like most about this town?
- What method of relaxation do you find most enjoyable?
- Why are you competing?
- Tell me about yourself.
- Are you superstitious?
- If you were expecting 8 guests for dinner and you burned the roast, what would you do?
- What do you think of women running for President?
- If you had a choice between fame and fortune, which would you choose and why?
- Do you feel that winning a pageant is the most important part of competition?
- Would you rather entertain friends or be entertained by friends?
- What do you consider the hallmarks of being a good neighbor?
- How do you behave around disabled individuals?
- How do you handle a tactless person who makes his prejudices known in social situations?
- What is the most unusual thing about your family?
- What is your most unforgettable experience?
- If you were to win, what's the first thing you'd say if someone shoved a mike in your hand?
- Some people claim Americans are preoccupied with winning. How important is winning to you?
- Only 20% of eligible voters under 25 vote. Why is that?
- What do you think it's going to take this country to elect a woman

President?

- Do you believe American youth are more interested in social issues or status issues?
- What is the biggest challenge facing the working woman today?
- What qualities would you look for in the man you would marry?
- What accomplishments are you proudest of?
- If you were a judge on this panel what qualities would you look for when selecting the Queen?

Appendix C

Pageant Books, Tapes, Magazines, and Newsletters

Books

Producing Beauty Pageants: A Director's Guide
by Anna Stanley
P.O. Box 1648
San Diego, CA 92118
(619) 437-4000

Becoming A Beauty Queen
by Barbara Peterson Burwell & Polly Peterson Bowles

The Miss Universe Beauty Book
by Susan Duff

The Cost of A Crown
by Nancy Carr
P.O. Box 15789
Durham, NC 27704-0789

The Beauty Pageant Manual
by Marie Leazer Farris and Verna Meer Glade
1862 Acuba Lane
Atlanta, GA 30345

Pageant Interview Questions and Techniques Volume I and II
What Should I wear for Interview That'll Look Great and Not Cost My Father A Fortune?
Life After Pageants Can Be a Career in Modeling
by Barbara Kelley

5305 Chemin de Vie
Atlanta, GA 30342
(404) 252-4924

Miss America Through The Looking Glass
by Nancie S. Martin

How To Be A Beauty Pageant Winner
by Marie Fenton Griffing

Southern Beauty
by Kylene Barker Brandon

The World of Miss Universe
by Ana Maria Cumba

Miss America, 1945
by Susan Dworkin

There She Is: The Life and Times of Miss America
by Frank Deford

A Bright Shining Place
by Cheryl Prewitt Salem with Kathryn Slattery
Health and Beauty Secrets
Choose to be Happy
You Are Somebody
by Cheryl Prewitt Salem
P.O. Box 701287
Tulsa, OK 74170

Tapes:

The Winning Look
Barbara Kelley
5305 Chemin de Vie
Atlanta, CA 30342

Be A Winner
Brooke Productions
7342 Haskell Ave., Suite 305
Van Nuys, CA 91406
(818) 786-4671

Winning A Pageant
Grewe Productions
P.O. Box 1131
Wheeling, WV 26003

How To Win Pageant Competitions
Lea and Lee Associates
9800 N. Campbell
K.C., MO 64155

TakeChargeofYourLife High Impact Aerobics
Cheryl and Friends Low Impact Aerobics
Cheryl Prewitt Salem
Infinity Video
P.O. Box 35035
Tulsa, OK 74153
1 (800) 331-3647

Magazines and Newsletters

Arizona Pageant Update
P.O. Box 9128
Phoenix, Arizona 85020
(602) 371-8779

Pageants & Talent
518 Madison Street
Huntsville, AL 35801
(800) 547-4176

Pageant Review
P.O. Box 446
Napoleon, Ohio 43545
(419) 592-8695

Pageantry
P.O. Drawer 3689
Baton Rouge, LA 70821
(504) 344-7628

Pageant Post
PO Box 643
Denham Springs, LA 70726
(504) 665-1033

Pageant Spotlight
3642 Bel-Pre Road, #24
Silver Spring, MD 20906
(301) 460-8574

The Competitive Edge
10922 Richards Court
Lenexa, KS 66210
(913) 469-6584

Pageant Peoples' Publication
201 U.S. 31 North
New Whitehead, IN 46184
(317) 535-9059

Pageant World
P.O. Box 568
Roseland, NJ 07068
(201) 228-5217

The Pageant Pace
P.O. Box 15789
Durham, NC 27704-0789
(919) 596-5301

Appendix D

Pageant Swimsuits and Shoes

Pageant Swimsuits

The Wior Corporation
Attn: The Crown Collection
2761 Fruitland Avenue
Los Angeles, CA 90058
(818) 846-3099

C P Annie Productions, Inc.
Attn: Cheryl's Winners!
P.O. Box 701287
Tulsa, OK 74170
(918) 495-6424

Pageant Swimsuit Designer

Ada Duckett
2204 Ravinia Dr.
Arlington, TX 76012
(817) 860-5399

Pageant Shoes

C P Annie Productions, Inc.
Attn: Pageant Shoes
P.O. Box 701287
Tulsa, OK 74170
(918) 495-6424

Appendix E

Musical Accompaniment Companies

Sound Choice
P.O. Box 2267
Charlotte, NC 28211
(704) 542-7616

Music Minus One
50 So. Buckhout St.
Irvington, New York 10533
(914) 591-5100

Pageant Tapes
C-6 Shore Dr.
Clinton, MS 39056
(601) 924-3544

Celebrity Series
International Productions
P.O. Drawer 3689
Baton Rouge, LA 70821
(504) 344-7628

Appendix F

Pageant Pointers

- Pack at least a week before the pageant.
- Be sure to include the shoes you plan on wearing.
- Include such items as safety pins, buttons, needle and thread.
- Check to see that your underclothes will function properly.
- If you are wearing hose, pack at least two pair.
- Do not bring anything of extreme value.
- Be punctual with applications, fees and registrations.
- Use good manners and be patient & helpful to others.
- Be alert and read all instructions.
- Refer to newsletters for any changes.
- Follow instructions during presentations.
- Be quiet during competition and speak softly.
- Be neat in the dressing areas and keep your own clothing and equipment together.
- Do not compete against others; only compete against yourself.

Put together your own checklist so you will be certain to remember all items. It is easier to rely on a checklist than your memory before pageant competition. When asked how important a pageant checklist is for contestants, Barbara Kelley responded, "I don't know how they do without it!"

Check to see that all outfits are secured at the seams and buttons and that your outfits have a secure fit. In a *Miss World* pageant *Miss Egypt* ran into misfortune when her dress fell down, leaving her bare from her ears to ber waist.

Pageant Checklist

Clothing
- Interview outfits (2)
- Evening gowns (2)
- Swimsuits (2)
- Costumes (if applicable)
- Pants/jeans
- Blouses
- Daytime outfits
- noncompetition swimsuit
- swimsuit coverup
- nylons (eight to ten)
- pajamas
- Bathrobe
- Nightgown
- socks

- brassiere (two or three regular and 1 strapless)
- panties (four or five)
- slips
- raincoat

Accessories
- jewelry
- purses
- shoes
- tote bag
- hat
- belts
- hair accessories

Medical Needs
- Band-Aids
- aspirin
- eye drops, vitamins, medications
- antacids
- analgesic pain relief rub
- petroleum jelly
- rubbing alcohol
- insect repellent
- spare contact lenses, contact lenses supply (if needed)

Beauty and Grooming Needs
- Blowdryers
- curling irons[1]
- electric makeup mirrow
- rollers
- extension cord[2]
- hairspray
- personal hygiene
- hair brush
- comb
- roller clips and bobby pins
- shampoo and conditioner
- hairpieces
- styling mousse
- cosmetics
- makeup tools
- cotton balls
- cotton swabs
- shower cap
- hand mirror
- hand and body lotions
- dental items
- deodorant
- manicure and pedicure items
- perfume
- razor and razor blades
- depilatory
- soap

Miscellaneous
- chaperone gift
- alarm clock
- photogenic pictures
- snack foods
- camera and film
- plastic baggies

---

1   Instead of having a dressing room with miles of curling iron cords, or for that matter a lack of outlets, butane curling irons are the solution for pageant competitors. They can be used anywhere without cords and plugs.

2   It is frustrating if curling irons or blow dryers won't reach the outlet.

- needle and thread
- safety pins
- sewing kit
- iron
- small ironing board
- contestants gifts (if necessary)
- state or national gift (if necessary)
- airline ticket (if Needed)
- spending money or travelers' checks
- adapter plugs (if traveling internationally)
- inflatable hangers[3]
- detergent
- washcloths
- umbrella
- books or magazines
- writing pens, address book, stationary, stamps
- sunglasses
- tackle box[4]

---

[3] If a garment is wrinkled, break out the inflatable hanger, hang the garment on it, close the shower curtains or door, hang the garment outside the shower, and then run the shower for 2-3 minutes until steam fills the room. Turn off shower and leave the garment hanging for 30 minutes.

[4] Jean Smith, Editor and Publisher of *Pageant Press*, says you can almost always spot the "Pageant Pro" — she is the one carrying the tackle box full of such items as needles and thread, super glue, scissors, safety pins, extra panty hose, shoe polish, curling, iron, bows, bobby pins, hair spray, makeup, aspirin, many of the items covered in the above checklist. These contestants plan their 'official' pageant gear and leave the articles intact for the next competition. They also keep a list of articles in the box that are removed so they are sure to replace them. The tackle box will stop the last minute searching before the next competition.

Appendix G

Professional Pageant Coaches and Posture Therapist

Pageant Coaches

Mary Francis Flood
304 Willeroy
Leland, MS 38756
(601) 686-7982

"The Winning Look"
Barbara Kelley
5305 Chemin De Vie
Atlanta, GA 30342

(404) 252-4924

The Competitive Edge Seminars
c/o Teddi Bankes-Domann and
Debra Fox
16909 W. 68th Street #261
Shawnee, KS 66217
(913) 469-6584

Posture Therapist

Bernice Danylchuck
Physio Dynamics
1399 Park Row
La Jolla, CA 92037
(619) 459-1180

Physio Dynamics
3655 Motor Avenue
Los Angeles, CA 90034
(213) 836-2556

Appendix H

National Pageant Addresses

Miss America
1325 Boardwalk
Boardwalk and Tennessee Ave.
Atlantic City, NJ 08401

Miss USA
Miss Teen USA
Miss Universe
6420 Wilshire Blvd., Suite 1500
Los Angeles, CA 90048

Miss Black America
Box 25668
Philadelphia, PA 19144

Mrs. America
2001 Wilshire Blvd, Suite 301
Santa Monica, CA 90403

Mother/Daughter Pageant
P.O. Box 2510
Hollywood, CA 90078

Miss Canada
Miss Teen Canada
c/o Cleo Productions
2 Bloor Street West, Suite 400
Toronto, Ontario
Canada M4W 3L2

English Leather Calendar Girl Pageant
Box 275527
Boca Raton, FL 33427

Miss Venus U.S.A.
240 Fairfield Avenue, Suite 213
Bridgeport, CN 06604

America's Junior Miss
P.O. Box 2786
Mobile, AL 36652

Miss Teenage America
c/o 'Teen magazine
8490 Sunset Blvd.
Los Angeles, CA 90069

Miss T.E.E.N.
P.O. Box 329
Long Prairie, MN 56347

Miss American Coed
Miss American Pre-Teen
3695 Wimbledon Dr.
Pensacola, FL 32504

Miss National Teen-Ager
215 Piedmont Ave., N.E.
Atlanta, GA 30308

Miss Teen All American
603 Scharder
Wheeling, WV 26003

The Junior America Show
11260 Chester Road, Suite 660
Cincinnati, OH 45246

Miss National Pre-Teen
214 Fifth Avenue
Lehigh Acres, FL 33970-1428

National Little/Junior Star
50 Beechwood Drive
Cranston, RI 02920

National Maid of Cotton
1918 North Parkway
Memphis, TN 38112

Miss Rodeo USA
3102 South Summitt Place
San Springs, OK 74063

Miss Rodeo America
Box L
McCall, ID 83638

Kids of America
P.O. Box 140339
Dallas, TX 75214

Celestial Beauty
P.O. Box 2668
Longview, TX 75606

America's Little Miss or Mr. Pageant
PO Box 2995
Louisville, KY 40229

Deep South Pageants
PO Box 45
Garrison, TX 75946

Miss Wheelchair America
600-25th Avenue South, St. 10
St. Cloud, MN 56301

Cinderella Scholarship Pageant
PO Drawer 3689
Baton Rouge, LA 70821

North American Youth Festival
954 Ecorse Road
Ypsilanti, MI 48198

Magazine Contests

Cosmo Girl Search
Cosmopolitan Beauty guide
224 West 57th St
New York, NY 10019

High School Cover Girl
Co-Ed Magazine
50 West 44th St.
New York, NY 10036

DID YOU BORROW THIS BOOK?

Become a Beauty Pageant Director!

Find out how you can reap the rich rewards of directing beauty pageants with this complete 384-page step-by-step guide to producing beauty pageants.

Among the topics covered in
Producing Beauty Pageants: A Director's Guide

- *Producing your first pageant with only $100*
- *How to get thousands of dollars worth of FREE advertising*
- *Registering hundreds of contestants into your pageants*
- *Tying major sponsors into your pageants*
- *Selling sub-sponsorship fees to prospective contestants and sub-sponsors*
- *Leading your pageant into big-league pageants*
- *Setting up a national system*
- *Airing your pageant on television*

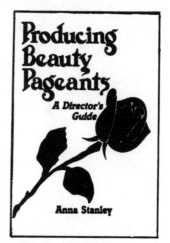

Producing Beauty Pageants

A Director's Guide

Anna Stanley